Shrinks

Shrinks
The Untold Story of Psychiatry

Jeffrey A. Lieberman, MD

with Ogi Ogas

(L)(B)

Little, Brown and Company
New York   Boston   London

Little, Brown and Company
Hachette Book Group
1290 Sixth Avenue, New York, NY 10104
littlebrown.com

First Edition: March 2015

Little, Brown and Company is a division of Hachette Book Group, Inc. The Little, Brown name and logo are trademarks of Hachette Book Group, Inc.

The publisher is not responsible for websites (or their content) that are not owned by the publisher.

The Hachette Speakers Bureau provides a wide range of authors for speaking events. To find out more, go to hachettespeakersbureau.com or call (866) 376-6591.

Copyright acknowledgments appear on p. 328.

ISBN 978-0-316-27886-7
Library of Congress Control Number: 2014956581

10 9 8 7 6 5 4 3 2 1

RRD-C

Printed in the United States of America

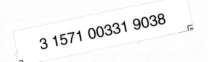

*For my parents, Howard and Ruth, who inspire me;
my wife, Rosemarie, and sons, Jonathan and Jeremy,
who support me; and my patients, who guide me.*

Contents

PART III
Psychiatry Reborn

The Brain is wider than the Sky,
For put them side by side
The one the other will contain
With ease — and You — beside.

The Brain is deeper than the sea,
For, hold them, Blue to Blue
The one the other will absorb
As Sponges, Buckets do.

The Brain is just the weight of God,
For, Heft them, Pound for Pound
And they will differ — if they do —
As Syllable from Sound.

— EMILY DICKINSON

Shrinks

What's Wrong with Elena?

Anyone who goes to a psychiatrist ought to have his head examined.

— SAMUEL GOLDWYN

A few years ago, a well-known celebrity—let's call him Mr. Conway—reluctantly brought his twenty-two-year-old daughter to see me. Elena had taken a leave of absence from Yale, Mr. Conway explained, because of issues surrounding a mysterious drop in her grades. Mrs. Conway nodded assent and added that Elena's slacking off stemmed from "a lack of motivation and low self-confidence."

In response to their daughter's perceived troubles, the Conways had hired a parade of motivational experts, life coaches, and tutors. Despite this pricey coterie of handlers, her behavior failed to improve. In fact, one tutor even volunteered (rather hesitantly, given Mr. Conway's celebrity) that "something is wrong with Elena." The Conways dismissed the tutor's concern as an excuse for his own incompetence and continued to look for ways to help their daughter "snap out of her funk."

They turned to naturopathic agents and meditation, and when those didn't help, they shelled out more money for hypnosis and acupuncture. In fact, they had done everything possible to avoid seeing a psychiatrist until "the incident."

While traveling uptown on the New York subway to meet her mother for lunch, Elena was accosted by a balding middle-aged man in a grimy leather jacket who coaxed her off the subway car. Without informing her mother, Elena abandoned the lunch appointment and accompanied the man to his seedy basement apartment on the Lower East Side. The man was in the kitchen preparing something alcoholic for her to drink when Elena finally answered a call from her frantic mother on her cell phone.

When Mrs. Conway learned where Elena was, she speed-dialed the police, who swooped in and carted her back to her parents. Elena didn't protest her mother's abrupt intervention; in fact, Elena didn't seem fazed by the incident at all.

As the Conways narrated these events in my Manhattan office, it was apparent that they loved their daughter and were genuinely concerned for her welfare. Having two sons of my own, I could easily empathize with their distress over the possible fate that could have befallen their daughter. Despite their concern, they made plain their doubts about the need for my services. After he sat down, the first thing Mr. Conway said was, "I gotta tell you, I really don't think she needs a shrink."

The profession to which I have dedicated my life remains the most distrusted, feared, and denigrated of all medical specialties. There is no anti-cardiology movement calling for the elimination of heart doctors. There is no anti-oncology movement protesting cancer treatment. But there is a large and vocal anti-psychiatry movement demanding that psychiatrists be downsized, reined in, or extirpated. As chairman of the psychiatry department at Columbia University, chief psychiatrist at the New York Presbyterian Hospital–Columbia University Medical Center, and past president of the American Psychiatric Association, I receive emails each week expressing pointed criticisms like these:

"Your bogus diagnoses exist merely to enrich Big Pharma."

"You take perfectly normal behaviors and call them illnesses to justify your existence."

"There is no such thing as mental disorders, only diverse mentalities."

"You quacks don't know what the hell you're doing. But you should know this: Your drugs destroy people's brains."

Such skeptics don't look to psychiatry to help *solve* mental health problems...they claim psychiatry *is* the mental health problem. All around the world, people have an abiding suspicion of "shrinks"—the most common epithet for the self-important charlatans believed to populate my profession.

I ignored the Conways' skepticism and began Elena's evaluation by taking her history, soliciting biographical and medical details from her parents. Elena, I learned, was the oldest and brightest of the Conways' four children and the one who seemed to hold the greatest potential. Everything in her life had been going great, her parents confided wistfully—until her sophomore year at Yale.

Open, gregarious, and popular during her freshman year, over a span of a few months Elena gradually stopped discussing her sorority life and romantic interests with her friends and parents. She adopted a strict vegetarian diet and became obsessed with the Kabbalah, believing its secret symbology would lead her to cosmic knowledge. Her attendance in class became erratic, and her grades dipped sharply.

At first, her parents were not worried by these changes. "You need to give kids space to find themselves," offered Mrs. Conway. "I sure marched to my own drummer when I was her age," agreed Mr. Conway. But Elena's parents finally became concerned after a phone call from Yale's student health services.

Elena had accused girls in her sorority of taunting her and stealing a gold bracelet. But when questioned by university administrators, Elena's sorority sisters denied any bullying— and they insisted they never saw the bracelet. They *had* noticed, on the other hand, that Elena's behavior had become increasingly strange. One of Elena's professors had even expressed concern over Elena's response to an exam question. When asked to explain James Joyce's stream of consciousness technique,

Elena wrote that Joyce's literary style was "a code with a special message to selected readers with wisdom implanted in their minds by the spiritual forces of the universe."

After that, the Conways requested a leave from school for Elena and enlisted private coaches and applied new age remedies until a friend recommended a popular Manhattan psychotherapist. This social worker was well known for promoting a decidedly nonmedical model of mental illness, pronouncing psychological issues as "mental roadblocks." As treatment, she favored a form of confrontational talk therapy of her own invention. She diagnosed Elena as suffering from a "self-esteem disorder" and began a series of expensive twice-weekly therapy sessions to help her remove her roadblocks.

After an entire year's worth of confrontational therapy produced no improvements, the Conways next turned to a holistic healer. He prescribed a purgative regimen, vegetarian diet, and meditative exercises, but despite his most creative efforts, Elena remained emotionally detached and mentally scattered.

Then the incident of the sleazy stranger's aborted abduction happened, forcing the Conways to confront the disconcerting fact that their daughter seemed oblivious to the dangers of going home with lecherous strangers. At this point their exasperated family physician implored them, "For Christ's sake, take her to a real doctor!" and they came to me.

Completing the interview with Elena's parents, I requested the opportunity to speak with their daughter privately. They left my office, and I was alone with Elena. She was tall, slender, and pale, with long blond hair that was tangled and unwashed. Earlier, as I was speaking with her parents, she had exhibited a demeanor of nonchalant distraction, like an idle cat. Now, as I addressed her directly, her gaze shifted randomly, as if she considered the lights in the ceiling to be more interesting than her interviewer.

Rather than feeling slighted, I felt genuine concern. I was familiar with this vacant and desultory gaze, which one colleague calls "fragmented attention." It suggested that Elena was attending to stimuli inside her mind rather than those unfolding in the room around her. Still contemplating Elena's distracted demeanor, I asked how she was feeling. She pointed to a photo on my desk of my wife and children. "I know those people," she replied, in a soft monotone like the whir of a ceiling fan. As I started to ask how she could know them, she interrupted. "I need to leave. I'm late for my appointment."

I smiled encouragingly. "This is your appointment, Elena. I'm Dr. Lieberman and your parents arranged this meeting to see if there is anything I might be able to do for you."

"Nothing's wrong with me," she replied in her flat, hushed voice. "I feel fine except my sisters keep making fun of me and messing with my artwork."

As I asked her about school and why she had left, she abruptly announced that she was no longer interested in school—she was on a quest to save the world by discovering the secret source of divine power. She believed God had placed angels in her parents' bodies to guide her on this sacred mission.

"Your secretary knows about it, too," Elena added.

"Why do you think that?"

"The way she smiled at me when I came in. It was a sign."

Such delusions, which psychiatrists classify as both "narcissistic" (relating incidental external events to one's self) and "grandiose" (imbuing mundane activities with transcendent purpose), are known as Schneiderian symptoms, after the German psychiatrist Kurt Schneider, who first described them in the 1940s as characteristic symptoms of psychosis. This initial constellation of behaviors and history strongly suggested a diagnosis of schizophrenia, the most severe and perilous of mental illnesses, and the illness I have studied for three decades.

I dreaded having to inform the Conways of this news, but at the same time I was shocked and saddened that this once lively girl may have been suffering with a highly treatable illness for three years while being repeatedly exposed to a series of useless remedies. Worse, by avoiding genuine psychiatric treatment, her parents had placed her at risk to very real dangers: First, her impaired judgment could have led her to make disastrous decisions. Second, we now know that if schizophrenia is left untreated it gradually induces irreversible brain damage, like the engine of a car driven without an oil change.

I invited Elena's parents back in. "So what's the verdict?" Mrs. Conway asked glibly, drumming her fingers on the chair. I told them I could not be completely sure until I had performed more tests, but it appeared likely their daughter had schizophrenia, a brain disorder affecting about 1 in 100 people that usually manifests in late adolescence or early adulthood. The bad news was that the illness was severe, recurrent, and incurable. The good news was that with the right treatment and sustained care there was an excellent chance she could recover and lead a relatively normal life, and even return to college. I knew the next part would be tricky: I looked Mr. and Mrs. Conway in the eyes and urged them to hospitalize their daughter immediately.

Mrs. Conway cried out in protest and disbelief. Her husband shook his head defiantly and fumed, "She doesn't need to be locked up in a *hospital*, for God's sake. She just needs to buckle down and get her act together!" I persisted, explaining that Elena needed continuous supervision and prompt treatment to safely restore her to sanity and avoid further hazards like the subway incident. Eventually they relented and agreed to admit her to the psychiatric unit of New York Presbyterian Hospital–Columbia University Medical Center.

I personally oversaw Elena's care. I ordered blood tests as

well as EEG, MRI, and neuropsychological assessments to rule out other causes of her condition, then prescribed risperidone, a very effective antipsychotic medication with only a modest potential for side effects. Meanwhile, in socialization groups, therapists helped her with her social skills. Cognitive therapy enhanced her attention and concentration. Guided instruction in the basic tasks of daily living aided her hygiene and appearance. After three weeks of medication and intensive care, cosmic symbols faded from her attention and Elena's natural personality started to shine through: She was cheerful and intelligent, with a playful sense of humor. She expressed embarrassment over her recent behavior and the strong desire to return to college and her friends in New Haven.

Her dramatic improvement was a testament to the power of modern psychiatry, and I couldn't wait to see Elena reunited with her parents. The Conways were delighted to get their daughter back, and I even saw Mr. Conway smile for the first time once he took in her transformation.

But when our treatment team met with the Conways to discuss Elena's discharge plan and the need for continuous outpatient care, they remained unconvinced that Elena's dramatic improvements were due to the medical treatment she had just received. Sure enough, a few weeks later I heard from the outpatient clinic that Elena had stopped showing up. I contacted the Conways and implored them to continue Elena's medical care, insisting that without it she was certain to relapse. While they thanked me for my help, they claimed they knew what was best for their daughter and would arrange for her treatment.

The truth is, if this had happened in the 1970s when I was in medical school and treating my very first patients, I might have sympathized with—or even shared—the Conways' aversion to psychiatrists. Back then, the majority of psychiatric institutions were clouded by ideology and dubious science, mired in a pseudomedical landscape where devotees of Sigmund Freud clung to every position of power. But the Conways were seeking treatment for their daughter in the twenty-first century.

For the first time in its long and notorious history, psychiatry can offer scientific, humane, and *effective* treatments to those suffering from mental illness. I became president of the American Psychiatric Association at a historic turning point in my profession. As I write this, psychiatry is finally taking its rightful place in the medical community after a long sojourn in the scientific wilderness. Buoyed by new research, new technologies, and new insights, psychiatry does not merely have the capacity to raise itself from the shadows but the obligation to stand up and show the world its revivifying light.

According to the National Institute of Mental Health, one in four persons will suffer from mental illness, and you are more likely to need services from psychiatry than from any other medical specialty. Yet far too many people—like the Conways—consciously avoid the very treatments now proven to relieve symptoms. Don't get me wrong; I would be the first to admit that psychiatry has earned much of its pervasive stigma. There's good reason that so many people will do everything they can to avoid seeing a psychiatrist. I believe that the only way psychiatrists can demonstrate just how far we have hoisted ourselves from the murk is to first own up to our long history of missteps and share the uncensored story of how we overcame our dubious past.

That's one reason I wrote this book: to provide an honest chronicle of psychiatry with all its rogues and charlatans, its queasy treatments and ludicrous theories. Until quite recently, authentic scientific triumphs were rare and bona fide psychiatric heroes rarer still. The history of sibling specialties like cardiology, infectious disease, and oncology are mostly narratives of steady progress punctuated by major leaps forward, while psychiatry's story consists mostly of false starts, extended periods of stagnation, and two steps forward and one step back.

But the full story of psychiatry is not just a dark comedy of fanciful gaffes. It is also a detective tale, propelled by three profound questions that have vexed and beckoned each successive generation of psychiatrists: What is mental illness? Where does it come from? And, most pressing for any discipline devoted to the Hippocratic oath, how can we *treat* mental illness?

From the start of the nineteenth century until the start of the twenty-first, each new wave of psychiatric sleuths unearthed new clues—and mistakenly chased shiny red herrings—ending up with radically different conclusions about the basic nature of mental illness, drawing psychiatry into a ceaseless pendulum swing between two seemingly antithetical perspectives on mental illness: the belief that mental illness lies entirely within the mind, and the belief that it lies entirely within the brain. Regrettably, no other medical specialty has endured such extreme volatility in its fundamental assumptions, and this volatility helped forge psychiatry's reputation as the black sheep of the medical family, scorned by other physicians and patients alike. But despite its many false leads and dead ends, the detective story of psychiatry has a gratifying finale in which its impenetrable mysteries have begun to be elucidated.

Over the course of this book, you'll learn about a handful of renegades and visionaries who bravely challenged the prevailing convictions of their time in order to elevate their embattled profession. These heroes declared that psychiatrists were not doomed to be shrinks but destined to be a unique class of physicians.

As a result of their pioneering triumphs, psychiatrists now understand that the successful treatment of mental illness requires us to embrace the mind and brain simultaneously. Psychiatry is like no other medical specialty; it transcends a mere medicine of the body to touch upon fundamental questions about our identity, purpose, and potential. It is grounded upon a wholly unique doctor-patient relationship: The psychiatrist often becomes privy to patients' private worlds and innermost thoughts—their most secret shames and most cherished dreams. The intimacy of this relationship places grave responsibility for the patient's welfare on the psychiatrist, a responsibility that psychiatrists have often failed to live up to—but no longer. The modern psychiatrist now possesses the tools to lead any person out of a maze of mental chaos into a place of clarity, care, and recovery. The world needs a compassionate and scientific psychiatry and I'm here to tell you, with little public fanfare, that such a psychiatry has arrived at last.

Let me share with you exactly what it took to get here...

Part I

The Story of Diagnosis

To name it is to tame it.
—Jeremy Sherman

Chapter 1

The Stepchild of Medicine: Mesmerists, Alienists, and Analysts

A sick thought can devour the body's flesh more than fever or consumption.

— GUY DE MAUPASSANT

Everything in nature communicates by a universal fluid. Nerves are the best conductors in the body for this universal magnetism and by touching these parts, you effect a happy turn of mind and bring on a radical cure.

— FRANZ MESMER, "DISSERTATION ON THE
DISCOVERY OF ANIMAL MAGNETISM"

Burning in the Air and the Soil

Abigail Abercrombie could no longer deny it: Something strange was happening to her, she just didn't know what. The year was 1946, and Abbey worked as a court stenographer for the Superior Court in Portland, Maine, a job demanding intense mental focus. Until recently, she had relished the daily challenge. But now, inexplicably, she was always distracted. She frequently misspelled words and sometimes omitted entire phrases in her transcriptions of testimony, all because she was preoccupied by the constant fear of having another "spell."

The spells had begun two months earlier, following her twenty-sixth birthday. The first one struck while she was shopping at a crowded grocery store. Without warning, all her senses screamed on high alert. She felt as if she couldn't breathe, and her heart pounded so hard she thought she must be dying. She rushed to the hospital, but after the doctors examined her they just patted her on the hand and told her that she was fine.

But she knew *something* wasn't right. Over the following month, she was blindsided by two more spells. Each time, for two or three minutes, her emotions seemed to go haywire, her heart raced, and she was filled with frantic terror. She began to wonder... *if the doctors say there is nothing wrong with my body, could something be wrong with my head?*

How does anyone really know if a disturbing psychic state is a genuine medical abnormality and not merely one of life's natural ups and downs? How do we recognize whether we—or someone we care about—is suffering from a pathological state of mind, rather than ordinary fluctuations in mental acuity and of high and low spirits? What *is* mental illness, exactly?

Oncologists can touch rubbery tumors, pulmonologists can peer through a microscope at strings of pneumonia bacteria, and cardiologists have little trouble identifying the yellowish plaques of artery-clotting cholesterol. Psychiatry, on the other hand, has struggled harder than any other medical specialty to provide tangible evidence that the maladies under its charge even exist. As a result, psychiatry has always been susceptible to ideas that are outlandish or downright bizarre; when people are desperate, they are willing to listen to any explanation and source of hope. Abbey didn't know where to turn—until she saw a story in the newspaper.

The story touted an impressive new treatment for emotional disturbances offered by the Orgone Institute, a mental health facility founded by a celebrated Austrian psychiatrist named Wilhelm Reich. Dr. Reich boasted impressive credentials from top medical institutions. He had been mentored by a Nobel laureate and served as an assistant director at the Vienna Psychoanalytic Polyclinic under the most famous psychiatrist of all, Sigmund Freud. Medical journals wrote favorably about his work, he had published several bestselling books, and even Albert Einstein endorsed his orgonomic treatments for emotional troubles — or so Reich claimed.

Hoping such an eminent physician might be able to finally diagnose what ailed her, Abbey paid a visit to Orgonon — a rural estate in Maine named in honor of Dr. Reich's research. To her delight, she was seen by Dr. Reich himself. With intense eyes and a high forehead crowned with a horizontal swath of unruly hair, he reminded her of the character Rotwang, the mad scientist in the 1927 film *Metropolis*.

"Are you familiar with orgones?" he asked her after she sat down.

When Abbey shook her head, Dr. Reich explained that all

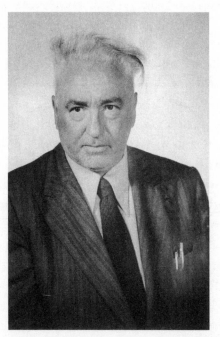

Wilhelm Reich (1897–1957), Freud disciple, psychoanalyst, originator of Orgone Theory. Photograph 1952. (© Bettmann/CORBIS)

mental illness—including her own condition, whatever it might be—stemmed from the constriction of orgones, a hidden form of energy uniting all of nature's elements. "This isn't a *theory*, the orgone is *burning* in the air and in the soil," insisted Dr. Reich, rubbing his fingers together. Physical and mental health, according to Dr. Reich, depended on the proper configuration of orgones, a term derived from the words "organism" and "orgasm."

Abbey nodded enthusiastically; this was exactly the kind of answer she had been looking for. "What you need," Dr. Reich continued, "is to restore the natural flow of orgones within your body. Fortunately, there is a way to do this. Would you like me to begin the treatment?"

"Yes, doctor."

"Please disrobe down to your underclothes."

Abbey hesitated. Every physician-patient relationship is founded upon a bedrock of trust, since we are granting the doctor unrestricted access to our body, from the blemishes on our skin to the depths of our bowels. But the psychiatrist-patient relationship runs deeper still, for we are entrusting the doctor with our *mind*—the very crux of our being. The psychiatrist calls upon us to reveal our thoughts and emotions—unveil our furtive desires and guilty secrets. The therapeutic relationship with a psychiatrist presumes that he is a trained expert and knows what he is doing, just like any orthopedist or ophthalmologist. But does the psychiatrist truly merit the same presumption of competence as other physicians?

Abbey hesitated for a moment but then recalled Dr. Reich's impressive credentials and medical training, slid out of her dress, carefully folded it, and placed it on the desk. Reich motioned for her to sit on a large wooden chair. She nervously sat down. The cool slats raised goose bumps on her bare legs.

The doctor approached her and gingerly began to touch her arms and shoulders, then moved down to her knees and thighs as if probing for tumors. "Yes, here—and here. Do you feel it? These are nexuses where your orgones are constricted. Please hold out your hand."

She obeyed. Without warning, he briskly smacked her arm just above her elbow, as if swatting a fly. Abbey cried out more from shock than pain. Dr. Reich smiled and raised his finger.

"There! You have *released* the energy locked inside! Don't you feel it?"

Each week for the next six months, Abbey returned to the Orgone Institute. During some of her visits, Dr. Reich used an "orgonoscope," an instrument that resembled a small brass telescope, to view the flow of orgone energy in her body, which—according to the doctor—was a bright electric blue. On other occasions, he instructed Abbey to strip down to her undergarments and squeeze into a telephone booth–sized box with a rubber hose dangling from her neck. This was an

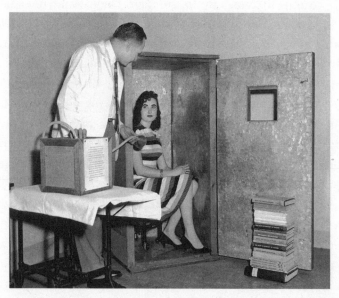

Orgone Accumulator, device used for Orgone Therapy. (© Food and Drug Administration/Science Source)

"orgone accumulator," which amplified Abbey's orgones and helped to reduce her anxiety.

Abbey gratefully accepted Dr. Reich's ministrations. She was not alone. People from all around the world sought help from Reich and his acolytes. His books were translated into a dozen languages, his orgone energy appliances were distributed internationally, and his ideas influenced a generation of psychotherapists. He was one of the most recognized psychiatrists of his era. But was the trust that Abbey placed in him justified?

In 1947, after Reich claimed his orgone accumulators could cure cancer, the FDA intervened. They soon concluded that his therapeutic devices and theory of orgone energy were a "fraud of the first magnitude." A judge issued an injunction banning all orgone devices and advertising. Reich—who genuinely believed in the power of orgones—was crushed. As the investigation progressed, former confidants reported that Reich was becoming increasingly paranoid and delusional; he believed that Earth was being attacked by UFOs, and he had taken to wandering through the Orgone Institute at night with his neck swathed in a bandana and a revolver at his waist, like some frontier gunfighter. During the subsequent trial for illegally selling orgone devices, the judge privately suggested that Reich might need his own psychiatrist. The jury found Reich guilty, the institute was shut down, and Reich was sentenced to prison. In 1957, he died in the Lewisburg Federal Penitentiary from heart failure.

We don't know exactly what Reich's patients felt when they learned that Wilhelm Reich's treatments were poppycock. But I can hazard a reasonable guess. Psychiatric chicanery, sadly, remains a problem to this very day, and I've encountered numerous patients who were treated by twenty-first-century charlatans. Not many things in life make you feel as violated as trusting your most intimate needs to a medical professional, only to have that trust betrayed through incompetence, deception, or delusion. I imagine Abbey repeating something a woman once told me upon discovering that her daughter's charismatic psychiatrist was trying to manipulate the twelve-year-old girl for his own purposes and turn her against her family: "He was a total phony. But how would we have ever known? We needed help, and everything about him seemed legitimate. How could anyone have known?"

As a psychiatrist myself, born while Wilhelm Reich was still treating patients, I have always been particularly troubled by one aspect of Reich's story: the failure of the psychiatric profession to expose one of their own as a fraud. Indeed, in the eyes of the public, the institution of psychiatry often seemed to endorse Reich's preposterous methods. Why was psychiatry unable to inform a public desperate for guidance that Reich's methods had no scientific basis whatsoever?

Unfortunately, unsound methods have never been far from the main currents of psychiatry, and leading psychiatric institutions have often credited techniques that were questionable, if not wholly inept. The sobering truth is that Wilhelm Reich is not a historical anomaly at all, but a discomfiting emblem of medicine's most controversial specialty.

Psychiatry's attempts to help the public distinguish evidence-based treatments from unsubstantiated fabrications have long been inadequate, and remain so today. You may wonder how thousands of educated intelligent people—teachers, scientists, and businesspeople, as well as court reporters—could have ever believed that an invisible network of orgasmic energy was the key to mental health. Yet even now, charlatans drawn from the ranks of professional psychiatry continue to dupe desperate and unsuspecting patients as the institutions of psychiatry passively stand by.

Daniel Amen, author of the popular *Change Your Brain* series of books and the star of PBS programs on the brain, might be the most recognized living psychiatrist. Joan Baez, Rick Warren, and Bill Cosby tout him, while the high-end motivational speaker Brendon Burchard once introduced Amen as "the number one neuroscience guy on the planet." Yet Amen's current fame rests entirely on spurious practices unproven by scientific research and rejected by mainstream medicine.

Amen suggests that by looking at images of the brain from SPECT scans (single photon emission computed tomography), he can diagnose mental illness—a practice that has more in common with skull-bump phrenology than modern psychiatry. "There is absolutely no evidence for his claims or practices," asserts Dr. Robert Innis, chief of molecular neuroimaging at the National Institute of Mental Health. In his opinion, "It is unscientific and unjustified, like using an unapproved drug." In an August 2012 *Washington Post* article, Dr. Martha J. Farah, director of the Center for Neuroscience & Society at the University of Pennsylvania, described Amen's technique more bluntly: "A sham." Dr. Amen also advocates the use of hyperbaric oxygen and markets his own brand of natural supplements as "brain enhancers"—treatments for which there is also no scientific evidence of efficacy.

Incredibly, current regulatory policies do not prevent someone like Amen from plying his SPECT mumbo jumbo. Even though every member of the governing board of the American Psychiatric Association regards his practice as medical flimflam, Amen continues unimpeded and largely unexposed. Even more frustrating to bona fide mental health practitioners, Amen brazenly claims that his unique methods are far ahead of the ponderous creep of mainstream psychiatry, which is rather like Bernie Madoff ridiculing the lower rate of return on a Fidelity mutual fund.

Just like Wilhelm Reich once was, Daniel Amen is cloaked

in a veneer of respectability that makes his techniques seem legitimate. If you were wondering how any of Reich's patients could have believed that stripping half-naked and climbing inside a strange orgone-collecting apparatus could enhance their mental health, you only need to consider the persuasive power of Amen's SPECT technique, which presents a striking parallel to orgone accumulators: Patients submit to the injection of radioactive agents into their veins and then dutifully place their heads in a strange gamma ray–collecting apparatus. The mystifying aura of SPECT, with its promise of cutting-edge science, seems as marvelous and bewitching as electric blue orgonomy. How can a layperson hope to distinguish between technologies that are scientifically proven and those conjured out of credible fancy?

To be sure, all medical specialties have suffered from their share of bogus theories, useless treatments, and misguided practitioners. Bleeding and colonic purges were once standard treatments for every malady from arthritis to the flu. Not so long ago, breast cancer was dealt with by radical mastectomies that gouged out most of the chest, including a woman's ribs. Even today, the FDA lists 187 oft-touted but apocryphal remedies for cancer. The use of antibiotics for colds is widespread, even though antibiotics have no effect on the viruses that cause colds, while useless arthroscopic surgery is too often performed for osteoarthritis of the knees. Bogus stem cell treatments for incurable neurologic illnesses like ALS and spinal cord injuries were the topic of a recent *60 Minutes* exposé. Sham treatments for autism abound, including vitamins, neutraceuticals, dietary supplements, stem cell injections, purges, and the removal of heavy metals from the body by chelation therapy. Patients trek across oceans in order to obtain exotic, expensive, and entirely worthless treatments for every imaginable disease. Even someone as intelligent as Steve Jobs was susceptible to far-fetched practices, delaying medical treatment of his pancreatic cancer in favor of "holistic medicine" until it was too late.

Nevertheless, psychiatry has trumpeted more illegitimate treatments than any other field of medicine, in large part because—until quite recently—psychiatrists could never agree on what actually constituted a mental disorder, much less how best to treat it. If each physician has his or her own definition of illness, then treatments become as varied as shoes, each season bringing a parade of new colors and fashions...and if you don't know *what* you are treating, then how can treatment ever be effective? Many of the most prominent names in the annals of psychiatry are better known for the dubiousness of their treatments than the good they achieved, despite their mostly charitable intentions: Franz Mesmer's animal magnetism, Benjamin Rush's "Bilious Pills," Julius Wagner-Jauregg's malaria therapy, Manfred Sakel's insulin shock therapy, Neil Macleod's deep sleep therapy, Walter Freeman's lobotomies, Melanie Klein's sexual orientation conversion therapy, and R. D. Laing's existential psychiatry.

I'm sorry to say that much of the responsibility for this state of affairs rests squarely on my profession. As the rest of medicine continues to enhance longevity, improve quality of life, and elevate expectations for effective treatments, psychiatrists are regularly accused of overprescribing drugs, overpathologizing normal behaviors, and spouting psychobabble. Many people harbor suspicions that even the best practices of twenty-first-century psychiatry might ultimately prove to be modern versions of Reich's orgonomy, spurious methods unable to relieve the suffering of individuals with bona fide illnesses—individuals like Abigail Abercrombie and Elena Conway.

Yet I would assert that today, my profession would help Abbey and Elena. Abbey would be confidently diagnosed as suffering from panic disorder without agoraphobia, a kind of anxiety disorder that is linked to dysfunction in neural structures in the medial temporal lobe and brain stem that control emotional regulation and fight-or-flight reactions. We would treat her condition with serotonin reuptake inhibiting medications (SRIs) and cognitive-behavioral therapy. With continued care, Abbey's prognosis would be quite optimistic, and she could expect to live a normal life with her symptoms controlled by treatment.

Elena had responded to her initial treatment well, and I believe that had she continued with the prescribed aftercare plan, she too would have had a good recovery and resumed her education and previous lifestyle.

But if I can be so confident about Abbey and Elena's diagnoses now, then why did psychiatrists stumble so egregiously in the past? To answer this, we must travel back more than two centuries, to psychiatry's origins as a distinct discipline of medicine. Because from the very moment of its birth, psychiatry has been a strange and wayward offspring: the stepchild of medicine.

A Medicine of the Soul

Since ancient times, physicians have known that the brain was the seat of thought and feeling. Any toga-clad medico could have told you that if the grayish-pink stuffing packed inside your skull was roughly thumped, as it often was in battle, you might go blind, talk funny, or drift into the comatose land of Morpheus. But in the nineteenth century, medical science in European universities began to combine the careful observation of a patient's abnormal behavior with refined autopsy dissections of their bodies after they died. Physicians peering through microscopes at brain sections and tissue of expired patients discovered, to their surprise, that mental disorders appeared to fall into two distinct categories.

The first category consisted of conditions where there was visible damage to the brain. While studying the brains of individuals who had suffered from dementia, doctors noticed that some looked smaller and were dotted with dark clumps of protein. Other physicians observed that patients who had abruptly lost movement in their limbs often had bulging blockages or ruddy stains in their brains (from strokes); on other occasions, glistening pink tumors were unearthed. The French anatomist Paul Broca analyzed the brains of two men with a combined spoken vocabulary of less than seven words (one man was named "Tan" because he relied on that single word for all of his communication). Broca discovered that each man had suffered a stroke in precisely the same location on the left frontal lobe. Gradually, many disorders became associated with readily identifiable "pathological signatures," including Parkinson's, Alzheimer's, Pick's, and Huntington's diseases.

Yet, when analyzing the brains of patients who had suffered from other kinds of mental disturbances, physicians failed to detect any physical abnormalities. No lesions, no neural anomalies—the brains of these patients had no features that distinguished them from the brains of individuals who never evinced behavioral dysfunction. These mysterious conditions formed the second category of mental disorders: psychoses, manias, phobias, melancholia, obsessions, and hysteria.

The discovery that some mental disorders had a recognizable biological basis—while others did not—led to the establishment of two distinct disciplines. Physicians who specialized exclusively in disorders with an observable neural stamp became known as *neurologists*. Those who dealt with the invisible disorders of the mind became known as *psychiatrists*. Thus, psychiatry originated as a medical specialty that took as its province a set of maladies that, by their very definition, had no identifiable physical cause. Appropriately, the term "psychiatry"—

coined by the German physician Johann Christian Reil in 1808—literally means "medical treatment of the soul."

With a metaphysical entity as its subject and raison d'être, psychiatry swiftly became a fertile ground for grifters and pseudoscientists. Imagine, for instance, if cardiology split into two distinct specialties: the "cardiologists" who dealt with the *physical* problems of the heart and the "spiritologists" who dealt with the *nonphysical* problems of the heart. Which specialty would be more vulnerable to fanciful theories and fraud?

Like the Bering Strait, the schism between the neurological brain and the psychiatric soul separated two continents of medical practice. Again and again over the next two centuries, psychiatrists would declare fraternity and equality with their neurological counterparts across the border, then just as abruptly proclaim liberty from them, insisting that the ineffable mind was the field of greater truth.

One of the earliest physicians who sought to explain and treat mental disorders was a German named Franz Anton Mesmer. In the 1770s he rejected the prevailing religious and moral accounts of mental illness in favor of a physiological explanation, making him arguably the world's first psychiatrist. Unfortunately, the physiological explanation he put forth was that mental illness could be traced to "animal magnetism"—invisible energy coursing through thousands of magnetic channels in our bodies—as could many medical illnesses.

Now, our modern minds might instinctively visualize these magnetic channels as networks of neurons with bioelectric impulses charging from synapse to synapse, but the discovery of neurons, let alone synapses, was still far off in the future. In Mesmer's time the notion of animal magnetism seemed as unfathomable and futuristic as if CNN announced today that we could now instantly travel from New York to Beijing using a teleportation machine.

Mesmer believed that mental illness was caused by obstructions to the flow of this animal magnetism, a theory eerily similar to the one Wilhelm Reich would espouse a century and a half later. Health was restored, claimed Mesmer, by removing these obstructions. When Nature failed to do this spontaneously, a patient could benefit from coming into contact with a potent conductor of animal magnetism—such as Mesmer himself.

By touching patients in the right places and in the right way—a pinch here, a caress there, some whispering in the ear—Mesmer claimed he could restore the proper flow of magnetic energy in their bodies. This therapeutic process was meant to produce what Mesmer referred to as a "crisis." The term seems appropriate. Curing an insane person, for example, required inducing a fit of unhinged madness. Curing a depressed person, one had to first render him suicidal. While this might seem counterintuitive to the minds of the uninitiated, Mesmer declared that his mastery of magnetic therapy allowed these induced crises to unfold under his control and without danger to the patient.

Here's a 1779 account of Mesmer treating an army surgeon for kidney stones:

> After several turns around the room, Mr. Mesmer unbuttoned the patient's shirt and, moving back somewhat, placed his finger against the part affected. My friend felt a tickling pain. Mr. Mesmer then moved his finger perpendicularly across his abdomen and chest, and the pain followed the finger exactly. He then asked the patient to extend his index finger and pointed his own finger toward it at a distance of three or four steps, whereupon my friend felt an electric tingling at the tip of his finger, which penetrated the whole finger toward the palm. Mesmer then seated him near the piano; he had hardly begun to play when my friend was

affected emotionally, trembled, lost his breath, changed color, and felt pulled toward the floor. In this state of anxiety, Mr. Mesmer placed him on a couch so that he was in less danger of falling, and he brought in a maid who he said was antimagnetic. When her hand approached my friend's chest, everything stopped with lightning speed, and my colleague touched and examined his stomach with astonishment. The sharp pain had suddenly ceased. Mr. Mesmer told us that a dog or a cat would have stopped the pain as well as the maid did.

Word of Mesmer's talent spread across Europe after he performed several remarkable "cures" using his powers of magnetism, such as restoring the sight of Miss Franziska Oesterlin, a friend of the Mozart family. Mesmer was even invited to give his opinion before the Bavarian Academy of Sciences and Humanities on the exorcisms carried out by a Catholic priest named Johann Joseph Gassner—a remarkable moment of irony, as one self-deluded faith healer was called upon to make sense of the methods of another. Mesmer rose to the occasion by proclaiming that while Gassner was sincere in his religious convictions and his exorcisms were indeed effective, they only worked because the priest possessed a high degree of animal magnetism.

Eventually, Mesmer made his way to Paris, where the egalitarian physician treated both wealthy aristocrats and commoners with his self-proclaimed powers of animal magnetism. As Mesmer's fame continued to grow, King Louis XVI appointed a scientific committee that included the visiting American scientist and diplomat Benjamin Franklin to investigate animal magnetism. The committee ultimately published a report debunking the methods of Mesmer and other practitioners of animal magnetism as nothing more than the power of imagination, though Franklin astutely observed, "Some think it will put an End to Mesmerism. But there is a wonderful deal of

Credulity in the World, and Deceptions as absurd, have supported themselves for Ages."

There is strong evidence that Mesmer really did believe in
the existence of preternatural magnetic channels. When he
became ill and lay on his deathbed, he waved off physicians
and repeatedly attempted to cure himself using animal
magnetism—to no avail. He perished in 1815.

Though Mesmer's fantastical theory did not survive into
the twentieth century, he was a psychiatric trailblazer in one
important respect. Before Mesmer, mental illness was widely
believed by physicians to have moral origins—according to
this view, the deranged had *chosen* to behave in a disreputable,
beastly manner, or at the very least, they were now paying the
piper for some earlier sin. Another common medical view was
that lunatics were born crazy, designed that way by the hand of
Nature or God, and that therefore there was no hope of treating them.

In contrast, Mesmer's peculiar theory of invisible processes
was actually quite liberating. He rejected both the determinis-
tic idea that certain individuals were born with mental illness
wired into their brains, and the sanctimonious notion that
mental illness signaled some kind of moral degeneracy, suggesting instead that it was the consequence of disrupted physiological mechanisms that could be treated medically. The
psychiatrist and medical historian Henri Ellenberger consid-
ers Mesmer the very first *psychodynamic* psychiatrist, a physician who conceptualizes mental illness as resulting from inner
psychic processes.

For a psychodynamic psychiatrist, the mind is more important than the brain, and psychology more relevant than biology. Psychodynamic approaches to mental illness would heavily
influence European psychiatry and eventually come to form
the central doctrine of American psychiatry. In fact, psychiatry
would swing back and forth for the next two centuries between

psychodynamic conceptions of mental illness and their intellectual opposite: *biological* conceptions of mental illness, holding that disorders arise from disruptions to the physiological operations of the brain.

After Mesmer, the first generation of physicians to embrace the term "psychiatrist" sought out other occult processes of the mind. Sometimes known as Naturalphilosophes, these early psychiatrists borrowed ideas from the Romantic movement in European arts and literature and pursued the irrational and covert forces in human nature, often believing in the power of a transcendent spirit and the inherent value of emotions. They rejected scientific experiments and direct clinical experience in favor of intuition and did not always draw a sharp line between mental illness and mental health. They often viewed madness as the result of a normal mind surrendering to the passionate and turbulent forces of the immortal soul.

The height of Romantic thought in early psychiatry found expression in the 1845 German textbook *Principles of Medical Psychology*, penned by a physician-poet-philosopher named Ernst von Feuchtersleben, who believed that "all branches of human research and knowledge are naturally blended with each other." Feuchtersleben's book was in such high demand that the publisher recalled the advance reading copies given free to universities and physicians so that they could be transferred to booksellers.

As you can imagine, a psychiatry of intuition and poetry did little to relieve the suffering of individuals assaulted by inner voices or immobilized by depression. Gradually, physicians came to recognize that focusing on unobservable processes shrouded within a nebulous "Mind" did not produce lasting change, or any change at all in patients with severe disorders. After decades of sailing through the foggy seas of psychic philosophizing, a new cohort of psychiatrists began to realize that this approach was steadily leading to their intellectual estrangement from the rest of medicine. These reactionary physicians condemned, often in harsh tones, the psychodynamic psychiatry of the Romanticists, accusing the Naturalphilosophes of "losing touch completely with practical life" as they plunged "into the mystico-transcendental realms of speculation."

By the mid-nineteenth century, a new generation of psychiatrists valiantly attempted to bridge the growing chasm between psychiatry and its increasingly respectable Siamese twin, neurology. This was the first wave of *biological psychiatry*, grounded in the conviction that mental illness was attributable to identifiable physical abnormalities in the brain. This movement was led by a German psychiatrist named Wilhelm Griesinger, who confidently declared that "all poetical and ideal conceptions of insanity are of the smallest value." Griesinger had been trained as a physician-scientist under the respected German pathologist Johann Schönlein, who was famous for establishing the scientific credibility of internal medicine by insisting that diagnoses should rely on two concrete pieces of data: (1) the physical exam and (2) laboratory analyses of bodily fluids and tissues.

Griesinger tried to establish the same empirical basis for psychiatric diagnosis. He systematically catalogued the symptoms of the inmates at mental asylums and then conducted pathological analyses of the inmates' brains after they died. He used this research to establish laboratory tests that could be performed on living patients, and crafted a structured interview and physical exam that could be used in conjunction with the laboratory tests to diagnose mental illness—or at least, that's what he hoped to achieve.

In 1867, in the first issue of his new journal, *Archives of Psychiatry and Nervous Disease*, Griesinger proclaimed, "Psychiatry has undergone a transformation in its relationship to the rest of medicine. This transformation rests principally on the realization that patients with so-called 'mental illnesses' are really individuals with illnesses of the nerves and brain. Psychiatry must therefore emerge from its closed off status as a guild to be an integral part of general medicine accessible to all medical circles."

This declaration of the principles of biological psychiatry inspired a new contingent of psychiatric pioneers who believed that the key to mental illness did not lie within an ethereal soul or imperceptible magnetic channels but inside the soft, wet folds of tissue in the brain. Their work gave rise to an enormous number of studies that relied heavily on the microscopic examination of postmortem brains. Psychiatrists trained in anatomy linked brain pathology to clinical disorders. (Alois Alzheimer, who identified the signature "senile plaques and neurofibrillary tangles" of the eponymous dementia, was a psychiatrist.) New brain-based theories were formulated, such as the proposal that mental disorders like hysteria, mania, and psychosis were caused by overexcited neurons.

Given these developments, you might have thought that the biological psychiatrists had finally positioned their profession on solid scientific ground. After all, there must be *some* discernible basis for mental illness in the brain itself, right? Alas, the research of the first generation of biological psychiatrists fizzled out like a Roman candle that soars into the sky without detonating. Despite making important contributions to neurology, none of the nineteenth-century biological theories of and research on mental illness ever found physical evidence to support them (other than the signature pathology of Alzheimer's disease), none led to eventual psychiatric breakthroughs, and none ultimately proved correct. No matter how carefully the biological psychiatrists pored over the fissures, gyri, and lobes of the brain, no matter how assiduously they scrutinized the slides of neural tissue, they could not find any specific and consistent aberrations indicative of mental illness.

Despite Griesinger's noble intentions, a reader of his *Archives of Psychiatry and Nervous Disease* would have no better understanding of mental illness than a reader of Mesmer's "Dissertation on the Discovery of Animal Magnetism." Whether you posited magnetic channels, a Universal Soul, or overexcited neurons as the source of mental illness, in the 1880s you would find precisely the same amount of empirical evidence to support your contention: none. Though brain research vaulted many nineteenth-century physicians into professorships, it produced no profound discoveries or effective therapies to alleviate the ravages of mental illness.

As the year 1900 fast approached, the conceptual pendulum began to swing again. Psychiatrists grew frustrated with the fruitless efforts of their biologically minded colleagues. One prominent physician dismissed biological psychiatry as "brain mythology," while the great German psychiatrist Emil Kraepelin (to whom we will return later) labeled it "speculative anatomy." Unable to find a biological basis for the illnesses within its province, psychiatry became ever more scientifically estranged from the rest of medicine. As if that wasn't bad enough, psychiatry had also become *geographically* estranged from the rest of medicine.

Caretakers for the Insane

Until the nineteenth century, the severely mentally ill could be found in one of two places, depending on their family's means. If the patient's parents or spouse had the good fortune to be a member of the privileged class, care could be administered at the family estate. Perhaps the patient could even be tucked away in the attic, like Mr. Rochester's mad wife in *Jane Eyre,* so that the affliction could be hidden from the community. But if the unfortunate soul came from a working-class family—or possessed heartless relatives—he would usually end up a homeless vagrant or in a residence of a very different sort: the asylum.

Every document of the era recording conditions inside pre-Enlightenment asylums makes them out to be wretched, filthy, teeming dungeons. (Horrific depictions of asylums would continue for the better part of the next two centuries, forming one of the most prominent themes of psychiatry and serving as endless fodder for journalistic exposés and causes for civil rights activism.) Inmates could expect to be chained, whipped, beaten with sticks, submerged in freezing water, or simply locked up in a cold, tiny cell for weeks at a time. On Sundays, they would often be displayed as freakish marvels before a gasping and taunting public.

The purpose of the earliest mental institutions was neither treatment nor cure, but rather the enforced segregation of inmates from society. For most of the eighteenth century, mental disorders were not regarded as illnesses and therefore did not fall within the purview of medicine, any more than the criminal behavior that landed a prisoner in a penitentiary. The mentally ill were considered social deviants or moral misfits suffering divine punishment for some inexcusable transgression.

One man was largely responsible for transforming asylums from prisons into therapeutic institutions of medicine and indirectly giving rise to a professional class of psychiatrists—a Frenchman by the name of Philippe Pinel. Pinel was originally a respected medical writer known for his gripping case studies. Then, in 1783, his life changed.

A close friend of Pinel's, a law student in Paris, came down with a form of madness that now would most likely be diagnosed as bipolar disorder. On one day the friend was filled with the exuberant conviction that he would soon become the most brilliant attorney in all of France; the next day he would plunge into despondency, begging for an end to his pointless life. Soon he believed that priests were interpreting his gestures and reading his mind. One night he ran off into the woods wearing nothing but a shirt and died from exposure.

This tragedy devastated Pinel and prompted him to devote the rest of his life to mental illness. In particular, he began investigating the operation of asylums, which he had consciously avoided when seeking care for his friend because of their notoriously wretched conditions. Before long, in 1792, he was appointed to head the Paris asylum for insane men at Bicêtre. He immediately used his new position to make major changes and took the unprecedented step of eliminating the noxious treatments of purging, bleeding, and blistering that were routinely used. He subsequently went on to free the inmates from their iron chains at the Parisian Hospice de la Salpêtrière.

Pinel eventually came to believe that the institutional setting itself could have beneficial effects on its patients, if properly managed. The German physician Johann Reil described how to go about establishing one of the new Pinel-style asylums:

> One might start by choosing an innocuous name, situate it
> in a pleasant setting, midst brooks and lakes, hills and fields,
> with small villas clustered about the administration build-
> ing. The patient's body and his quarters were to be kept
> clean, his diet light, neither spirituous nor high seasoned. A
> well-timed variety of amusements should be neither too long
> nor too diverting.

This was a far cry from the bleak prisons for undesirables that constituted most other asylums. This started what became known as the asylum movement in Europe and later spreading to the United States. Pinel was also the first to argue that the routine of the asylum should foster the patients' sense of stability and self-mastery. Today, most psychiatric inpatient units, including the ones here at the New York Presbyterian Hospital–Columbia University Medical Center, still employ Pinel's concept of a routine schedule of activities that encourages structure, discipline, and personal hygiene.

After Pinel, the conversion of mental institutions into places of rest and therapy led to the formal establishment of psychiatry as a clearly defined profession. To transform an asylum into an institution of therapeutic humanity rather than of cruel incarceration required doctors who specialized in working with the mentally ill, giving rise to the first common appellation for the psychiatrist: *alienist.*

Alienists were given their nickname because they worked at asylums in rural locales, far removed from the more centrally located hospitals where the alienists' medical colleagues worked and socialized and tended to physical maladies. This geographical separation of psychiatry from the rest of medicine has persisted into the twenty-first century in a variety of ways; even today, there are still *hospitals* and *mental hospitals,* though fortunately the latter are a dying breed.

Throughout the nineteenth century, the vast majority of psychiatrists were alienists. While the various psychodynamic and biological theories of mental illness were usually proposed and debated in the halls of academia, these ideas for the most part had little impact on the day-to-day work of the alienists. To be an alienist was to be a compassionate caretaker rather than a true doctor, for there was little that could be done to mitigate the psychic torments of their charges (though they did minister to their medical needs as well). All the alienist could hope to accomplish was to keep his patients safe, clean, and well cared for—which was certainly far more than had been done in previous eras. Still, the fact remained that there was not a single effective treatment for mental illness.

As the nineteenth century came to a close, every major medical specialty was progressing by leaps and bounds—except for one. Increasingly intricate anatomical studies of human cadavers produced new details of liver, lung, and heart pathologies—yet there were no anatomical drawings of psychosis. The invention of anesthesia and sterile techniques enabled ever more complex surgeries—but there was no operation for depression. The invention of X-rays allowed physicians the near-magical power to peer inside living bodies—but even Roentgen's spectacular rays failed to illuminate the hidden stigmata of hysteria.

Psychiatry was exhausted by failure and fragmented into a menagerie of competing theories regarding the basic nature of mental illness. Most psychiatrists were alienists, alienated from both their medical colleagues and the rest of society, keeping watch over inmates who had little hope of recovery. The most prevalent forms of treatment were hypnosis, purges, cold packs, and—most common of all—firm restraints.

Karl Jaspers, a renowned German psychiatrist turned existentialist philosopher, recalled the mood at the turn of the century: "The realization that scientific investigation and therapy were in a state of stagnation was widespread in psychiatric clinics. The large institutions for the mentally ill were more magnificent and hygienic than ever, but despite their size, the best that was possible for their unfortunate inmates was to shape their lives as naturally as possible. When it came to *treating* mental illness, we were basically without hope."

Nobody had the slightest idea why some patients believed God was talking to them, others believed that God had abandoned them, and still others believed they *were* God. Psychiatrists yearned for someone to lead them out of the wilderness by providing sensible answers to the questions, "What causes mental illness? And how can we treat it?"

A "Project for a Scientific Psychology"

In W. H. Auden's poem "In Memory of Sigmund Freud," he writes of the difficulty of understanding Freud through our modern eyes: "He is no more a person now but a whole climate of opinion." It's a pretty safe bet that you've heard of Freud and know what he looks like; his Edwardian beard, rounded spectacles, and familiar cigar make him the most famous psychiatrist in history. The mention of his name instantly evokes the phrase, "So tell me about your mother." It's also quite likely that you have an opinion on the man's ideas—and, I'd wager, an opinion shading into skepticism, if not outright hostility. Freud is often maligned as a misogynist, a self-important and domineering phony, or a sex-obsessed shrink endlessly probing people's dreams and fantasies. But, to me, he was a tragic visionary far ahead of his time.

In the pages of this book we will encounter many psychiatric luminaries (like Nobel laureate Eric Kandel) and psychiatric frauds (like orgonomist Wilhelm Reich). But Sigmund Schlomo Freud stands in a class of his own, simultaneously psychiatry's greatest hero and its most calamitous rogue. To my mind, this apparent contradiction perfectly captures the paradoxes inherent in any effort at developing a medicine of mental illness.

I doubt I would have become a psychiatrist if it weren't for Freud. I encountered the Austrian physician for the first time as a teenager when I read his most celebrated work, *The Interpretation of Dreams*, in a freshman psychology course. There was something about Freud's theory and the manner in which he communicated it that seemed to unlock the great mysteries of human nature—and resonated with my own efforts to understand myself. I thrilled to such sentences as: "The conscious mind may be compared to a fountain playing in the sun and falling back into the great subterranean pool of subconscious from which it rises."

There's a common phenomenon among medical students known as "intern's syndrome": studying the list of symptoms for some new ailment, the student realizes—lo and behold—she herself must be afflicted with diphtheria, or scabies, or multiple sclerosis. I experienced a similar reaction with my initial exposure to Freud. I began to reinterpret my behavior through Freud's theories with a sudden rush of apparent insight. Did I argue so often with my male professors because of a repressed Oedipal conflict with my father over winning my mother's attention? Was my room messy because I was stuck in the anal stage of psychosexual development as a consequence of my mother making me wear a diaper to nursery school?

While I may have indulged in overly elaborate interpretation of trivial behaviors, Freud did teach me the invaluable lesson that mental phenomena were not random events; they were determined by processes that could be studied, analyzed, and, ultimately, illuminated. Much about Freud and his influence on psychiatry and our society is paradoxical—revealing insights into the human mind while leading psychiatrists down a garden path of unsubstantiated theory. Most people forget that Freud was originally trained as a hard-nosed neurologist who advocated the most exacting standards of inquiry. His 1895 work *Project for a Scientific Psychology* was intended to educate physicians about how to approach psychiatric issues from a rigorous scientific perspective. He trained under the greatest neurologist of the age, Jean-Martin Charcot, and—like his mentor—Freud presumed that future scientific discoveries would clarify the underlying biological mechanisms responsible for thought and feeling. Freud even presciently diagrammed what may be one of the earliest examples of a neural network, depicting how systems of individual neurons might communicate with one another to learn and perform computations, foreshadowing the modern fields of machine learning and computational neuroscience.

While Wilhelm Reich frequently made public claims that Albert Einstein endorsed his ideas about orgonomy, in actuality, Einstein considered Reich's ideas ludicrous and demanded that he stop using his name to market his products. But the great physicist had a very different attitude toward Freud. Einstein respected Freud's psychological acumen enough to ask him, shortly before World War II, to explain man's capacity for warfare, requesting that Freud "might bring the light of [his] far-reaching knowledge of man's instinctive life to bear upon the problem." After Freud responded with a dissertation upon the subject, Einstein publicly endorsed Freud's views and wrote back to Freud, "I greatly admire your passion to ascertain the truth."

Freud's pioneering ideas on mental illness were initially sparked by his interest in hypnosis, a popular nineteenth-century treatment that originated with Franz Mesmer. Freud was captivated by the uncanny effects of hypnosis, especially the mysterious phenomenon whereby patients accessed memories that they could not recall during their normal state of awareness. This observation eventually led him to his most celebrated hypothesis: that our minds contain a hidden form of awareness that is inaccessible to our waking consciousness. According to Freud, this *unconscious* part of the mind was the mental equivalent of a hypnotist who could make you stand up or lie down without your ever realizing why you had done so.

These days we take the existence of the unconscious for granted; it strikes us as so obvious a phenomenon that it almost seems ridiculous to credit a single person with "discovering" it. We casually use terms like "unconscious intention," "unconscious desire," and "unconscious resistance" and tip our hat to

Sigmund by referring to "Freudian slips." Modern brain and behavioral scientists also take the unconscious as a given; they embrace the unconscious in such concepts as implicit memory, priming, subliminal perception, and blindsight. Freud called his counterintuitive theory of an unconscious mind *psychoanalytic theory*.

Freud dissected the mind into various components of consciousness. The primal *id* was the voracious source of instincts and desires; the virtuous *superego* was the voice of conscience, a psychological Jiminy Cricket proclaiming, "You can't do that!"; the pragmatic *ego* was our everyday consciousness, called upon to mediate between the demands of the id, the admonitions of the superego, and the reality of the world outside. According to Freud, humans are only partially privy to the workings of their own minds.

Freud drew upon this novel conception of the mind to propose a new psychodynamic definition of mental illness that would shift the course of European psychiatry, then come to reign over American psychiatry. According to psychoanalytic theory, every form of mental illness could be traced to the same root cause: conflicts between different mental systems.

For example, Freud would say that if you unconsciously wished to have sex with your married boss, but consciously knew that doing so would lead to all kinds of trouble, this would produce a psychic conflict. Your conscious mind would first try to deal with the conflict through straightforward emotional control ("yes, I think my boss is attractive, but I'm mature enough to not give in to those feelings"). If that failed, your conscious mind would try to resolve the conflict using psychological sleights of hand that Freud called *defense mechanisms*, such as *sublimation* ("I think I will read some erotic stories about forbidden affairs") or *denial* ("I don't think my boss is attractive, what are you talking about?!"). But if this psychic clash was too intense for your defense mechanisms to manage, it might trigger hysteria, anxiety, obsessions, sexual problems, or—in extreme cases—psychosis.

Freud's broad term for all mental disturbances caused by unresolved psychic conflicts that affected people's emotions and behavior but did not cause them to lose touch with the reality of the external world was *neurosis*. Neurosis would become the foundational concept within psychoanalytic theory for understanding and treating mental illness—and the most influential clinical concept in American psychiatry throughout most of the twentieth century, until 1979, when the seminal revision of psychiatry's system of diagnosis was completed and neurosis would become the subject of a climactic battle over American psychiatry's soul.

But in the early 1900s, Freud had no tangible evidence whatsoever of the existence of the unconscious or neurosis or any of his psychoanalytical ideas; he formulated his theory entirely from inferences derived from his patients' behaviors. This may seem unscientific, though such methods are really no different from those used by astrophysicists positing the existence of dark matter, a hypothetical form of invisible matter scattered throughout the universe. As I write this, nobody has ever observed or even detected dark matter, but cosmologists realize that they can't make sense of the movements and structure of the observable universe without invoking some mysterious, indiscernible *stuff* quietly influencing everything we can see.

Freud also provided far more detailed and thoughtful reasoning about mental illness than had been offered as the basis for any prior psychiatric theories. In particular, he considered neurosis a neurobiological consequence of Darwinian processes of natural selection. Human mental systems evolved to support our survival as social animals living in communities where we needed to both cooperate and compete with other members of our species, Freud argued. Therefore, our mind evolved to repress certain selfish urges in order to facilitate essential cooperation. But sometimes our cooperative and competitive urges conflict with one another (if we become sexually attracted to our boss, for example). This conflict is what produces psychic discord, and if the discord is not resolved, Freud postulated, it could unbalance the natural operation of the mind and create mental illness.

Critics of Freud often wonder why sex figures so prominently in his theories, and though I agree that his overemphasis on sexual conflict was one of his most glaring mistakes, he had a rational explanation for it. Since sexual urges are essential for reproduction and contribute so heavily to an individual's evolutionary success, Freud reasoned that they were the most potent and selfish Darwinian urges of all. So when we try to repress our sexual desires, we are going against millions of years of natural selection—thereby generating the most intense psychic conflict of all.

Freud's observation that sexual desires can often lead to inner conflicts certainly resonates with most people's experiences. Where he went astray, to my mind, was in presuming that because our sexual urges are so strong they must make their way into every single one of our decisions. Neuroscience, as well as casual introspection, tells us otherwise: that our desire for wealth, acceptance, friendship, recognition, competition, and ice cream are all independent and equally real impulses, not merely lust in costume. Although we may be creatures of instinct, our instincts are not solely, or even mostly, sexual.

Freud described several examples of neuroses in his celebrated case studies, including that of Dora, the pseudonym for a teenage girl who lived in Vienna. Dora was prone to "fits of coughing accompanied by a loss of voice," particularly when talking about her father's friend Herr K. Freud interpreted Dora's loss of speech as a kind of neurosis he termed a "conversion reaction." Herr K. had apparently made a sexual advance to the underage Dora, pressing himself against her. When Dora told her father about his friend's behavior, he did not believe her. At the same time, Dora's father was having a furtive affair with Herr K.'s wife, and Dora, who knew of their romantic liaison, thought that her father was actually encouraging her to spend more time with Herr K. as a way of giving himself greater opportunities with Herr K.'s wife.

Freud interpreted Dora's conversion disorder as resulting from the unconscious conflict between wanting to maintain harmonious relations with her father and wanting him to believe her about his friend's repulsive behavior. Dora's mind, according to Freud, "converted" the desire to tell her father about his friend's sexual aggressiveness into muteness in order to preserve her relationship with him.

Conversion disorders had been recognized for a long time before Freud gave them a name, but he was the first to offer a plausible explanation of the phenomenon—in Dora's case, explaining her inability to talk as an attempt by her conscious mind to repress a truth about something that might make her father angry at her. While Freud's analysis of Dora's case becomes increasingly far-fetched and insensitive—he eventually suggests that Dora was sexually attracted to both her father and Herr K., and we can't help but sympathize with Dora when she abruptly terminated her therapy with Freud—his core insight that certain kinds of abnormal behaviors can be traced to inner conflicts remains relevant to this day. In fact, I've encountered patients who seem to have stepped straight out of Freud's casebook.

Some years ago I was asked to examine a forty-one-year-old man named Moses who worked at a neighboring community hospital. All in all, Moses's life was fairly stable—except for the situation with his boss. Moses liked his boss, the chief of cardiology; after all, the man had promoted Moses into the comfortable position of chief division administrator. Moses felt he owed the man his loyalty since, as Moses saw it, his boss had single-handedly enabled his professional success. But at the time I started seeing him as a patient, Moses was beginning to understand the cost of this loyalty.

Moses's boss was embroiled in an intense battle with the hospital president over financial issues. During their angry skirmishes, Moses was often called upon by his boss to review financial data and compile reports. Gradually, Moses began to piece together a troubling picture: His boss was intentionally misrepresenting the division's finances to the president. Worse, it was becoming increasingly clear that his boss was covering up a string of deceptive and possibly illegal financial transactions.

Moses was horrified. He knew that the hospital administration would eventually discover his boss's secret—and Moses himself would share the blame, since everyone would presume he had known about his boss's transgression and was therefore complicit in it. He was torn between his loyalty to the man who gave him his job and the desire to behave honestly. As the confrontation between his boss and the president escalated, Moses's anguish increased until he reached his breaking point.

One day at work, Moses abruptly began to have difficulty speaking. Soon he was stuttering. He became confused and disoriented. By the end of the day, he had become entirely mute. He opened his mouth but no sound came out, only guttural rasps. This disturbing change in behavior prompted his colleagues to whisk him off to the emergency room.

The doctors immediately presumed Moses had experienced a stroke or seizure, the usual suspects when someone suddenly becomes confused and unable to speak. They ordered a complete neurological workup, including a CT scan and an EEG. To their surprise, the tests came back completely normal. Without any evidence of a physiological abnormality, the problem was presumed to be psychiatric, and Moses was referred to me.

At first, I suspected some form of malingering—perhaps he was faking symptoms to get sick leave or collect disability insurance—but there was no evidence to support this hypothesis. Moses's muteness extended to all areas of his life, even when he was home with family and friends. I recommended that he be placed on medical leave and scheduled a follow-up visit. When he arrived at my office, I told him that I would like to perform a diagnostic procedure called an amytal interview. This was an old procedure that involved administering a moderate dose of a short-acting barbiturate intravenously. It relaxes and disinhibits the patient and thus can act as a kind of truth serum. Moses nodded his consent.

I brought him into a treatment room, placed him on a gurney, and filled a syringe with amobarbital. Inserting the needle into his vein, I slowly began to inject the liquid medication. In less than a minute he began to speak, at first in a garbled and childlike fashion, then clearly and coherently. He explained the jam he was in at work and declared that he didn't know what to do. After recounting all the details of his dilemma, he abruptly fell asleep. When he awoke a short while later, he was once again unable to speak, but the "truth serum" had confirmed my guess: His muteness was a conversion reaction. (The latest edition of the *Diagnostic and Statistical Manual of Mental Illness* contains a formal diagnosis for conversion disorders that is largely based on Freud's conception.)

After missing work for a few weeks, Moses was informed that he was being transferred to another department and would no longer work for his former boss or be responsible for the cardiology division's finances. Within a few days of this news, Moses fully regained his ability to speak. Freud, I think, would have been pleased with the outcome.

*   *   *

By defining mental illness as conflicts between unconscious mechanisms—conflicts that could be identified, analyzed, and even eliminated—Freud provided the first plausible means by which psychiatrists could understand and treat patients. The appeal of Freud's theory was enhanced by his spellbinding skills as a speaker and his lucid and compelling writing. Surely this was the leader that psychiatry had been yearning for, someone who could boldly lead the field into the new century and back into the good graces of their medical brethren.

Instead, Freud ended up leading psychiatry into an intellectual desert for more than a half century, before eventually immersing the profession into one of the most dramatic and public crises endured by any medical specialty. How did this happen? Part of the answer lies with individuals like Elena Conway and Abigail Abercrombie—patients suffering from debilitating illnesses.

Part of the answer lies within Freud himself.

Chapter 2

Down the Garden Path: The Rise of the Shrink

Psychiatry enables us to correct our faults by confessing our parents' shortcomings.

— LAURENCE PETER

Sigmund Freud was a novelist with a scientific background. He just didn't know he was a novelist. All those damn psychiatrists after him, they didn't know he was a novelist either.

— JOHN IRVING

A Coffee Klatch

Like the smart phone, Freud's exciting new conception of the mind was embraced so universally that it became difficult to remember what life was like before it arrived. Freud made mental illness seem fresh, comprehensible, and intriguing. But unlike smart phones—which were adopted rapidly after their introduction—the influence of psychoanalytic theory spread slowly.

A better comparison for Freud's theories might be video teleconferencing, a technology that was completely shrugged off by the public when it was first introduced in the 1970s, though it finally caught on decades later on the heels of the Internet and mobile devices. So how did psychoanalytic theory grow from the idiosyncratic conjectures of an unknown neurologist to become as commonplace as Skype? It all started with an evening coffee klatch.

A Small Circle of Colleagues

In the autumn of 1902, Freud sent postcards to four local physicians, inviting them to his row house apartment in the Berggasse district of Vienna, a drab, uninspiring middle-class Jewish neighborhood. One postcard read: "A small circle of colleagues and supporters would like to give me the great pleasure of coming to my place one evening a week to discuss topics of interest to us in psychology and neuropsychology. Would you be so kind as to join us?"

Freud's book *The Interpretation of Dreams* had been published less than two years earlier, but the book hadn't made much of a splash, or even a ripple. Its very modest print run of six hundred copies was languishing at booksellers. Nevertheless, a handful of physicians were sufficiently intrigued by Freud's decryption of the workings of the mind to strike up an admiring correspondence with him. One of these early enthusiasts was Wilhelm Stekel, a vivacious and outspoken general physician and a writer of plays and poems. Stekel volunteered to become one of the very first patients to be psychoanalyzed by Freud and went on to become a psychoanalyst himself. In the midst of his therapy, Stekel advanced a history-altering recommendation: Freud should hold a discussion group to talk about his ideas.

The fact that exactly four people were invited to Freud's first coffee klatch hints at the deflating initial lack of interest in his work. Stekel was the first invitee. Two others were Freud's childhood friends (Max Kahane and Rudolf Reitler). The fourth was Alfred Adler, the only recruit with any meaningful influence in the medical field at the time. Adler was a Socialist physician who enjoyed the camaraderie of groups and felt completely at home among the working classes. He dressed and carried himself like a blue-collar laborer and had published an occupational health book for tailors.

Together with Freud, these four men formed the nucleus of what would eventually become an international movement. The group decided to meet in Freud's dark and tiny living room every Wednesday evening, prompting the name for their little clique: the Wednesday Psychological Society. Despite these humble beginnings, according to Stekel, the earliest meetings featured "complete harmony among the five, no dissonances; we were like pioneers in a newly discovered land, and Freud was the leader. A spark seemed to jump from one mind to the other, and every meeting was a revelation."

The society soon began to attract nonphysicians, including an opera producer, a bookseller, an artist, and a novelist. Meetings followed a prescribed routine. The men would gather around an oblong table in Freud's Victorian-styled parlor at 8:30 p.m. sharp. Presentations commenced at 9:00 p.m. Names were drawn from an urn to determine the order of the speakers. After the formal talks, there was fifteen minutes of socializing. Cigars and cigarettes were laid out on a table and smoked in great quantities. Black coffee and cakes were served and hungrily devoured. Max Graf, an Austrian musicologist who joined the society in 1903, described the mood: "There was the atmosphere of the founding of a religion in that room, and Freud himself was its new prophet."

The last and decisive word of each meeting was left to Freud. The minutes of one meeting, during which the members debated the role of incest in neurosis, report how Freud closed the session by "telling of a disguised form of the dream of incest with the mother. The dreamer is in front of the entrance to a house. The dreamer goes inside. He has the vague recollection of having been in there once before. It is the mother's vagina, for this is the place where he has been once before."

Initially, meetings of the Wednesday Psychological Society mainly focused on the theoretical and social implications of Freud's ideas. But the members of the society soon became eager to apply this new theory to alleviate the suffering of those who were mentally disturbed. Since Freud believed that most psychiatric problems resulted from inner psychic conflicts, he developed an ingenious and highly original method to relieve these conflicts.

Freud's "talking cure," as he called it, derived from two distinct forms of therapy he had been exposed to during his early career. The first was hypnosis. As part of his neurological fellowship under Jean-Martin Charcot in 1885, Freud learned to use hypnosis with patients suffering from hysteria, which at the time was a vaguely defined condition consisting of volatile and unmanageable emotions. Freud marveled at how hysterical symptoms often seemed to dissipate after a hypnotic session. He gradually came to believe that it might be possible to adapt hypnosis into a more methodical form of talk therapy (or *psychotherapy*, in the vocabulary of psychiatry).

Freud's talking cure also had roots in the methods of Viennese physician Josef Breuer, who mentored the young Freud in the late 1880s and set him up with his first medical practice. As Breuer's protégé, Freud observed that when one of Breuer's young female patients (known to history as Anna O) rambled aimlessly to Breuer about whatever thoughts came into her mind, her psychiatric symptoms diminished or disappeared. Anna referred to this process of uninhibited speech as "chimney sweeping," while Breuer called it the "cathartic method." Freud combined Charcot's hypnosis and Breuer's cathartic method with his evolving psychoanalytic theory to fashion the first systematic form of psychotherapy, which he dubbed *psychoanalysis*.

Psychoanalysis was conceived as a method of probing

patients' unconscious minds to identify their hidden conflicts. During psychoanalysis, Freud encouraged patients to free-associate, speaking about anything that came to mind. Since Freud viewed dreams as an invaluable source of information about unconscious conflicts (he famously called them the "royal road to the unconscious"), he also encouraged patients to share details of their dreams during psychoanalysis. The great benefit of psychoanalysis, Freud insisted, was the fact that hypnosis worked on only about one-third of patients, while psychoanalysis worked on everyone.

Freud's psychoanalytic method came to define many of the traditional forms of psychiatrist-patient interactions that continue to this day, including frequent therapy sessions, the 45- or 50-minute session, guided communication with the patient, and a comfortable therapist's office with a couch or overstuffed armchair. Psychoanalysts usually sat behind their patients, a technique that was carried over from Freud's earliest days when he sat behind patients while hypnotizing them so that he could press their foreheads while solemnly urging them to remember events blocked from their consciousness.

The clinical practice of the unobservable therapist later acquired a theoretical justification through the concept of *transference*. During psychoanalysis, the therapist was to become a blank slate, remote and aloof and removed from view, in order to facilitate the patient's projection of past relationships onto the therapist. This was believed to induce the eruption of revelations from the unconscious, like submitting oneself to the Oracle of Delphi.

While contemporary psychiatrists no longer stay hidden from their patients' view, the Freudian concept of transference has endured as one of the cornerstones of modern psychotherapy and is taught to every psychiatric resident, clinical psychology grad student, and social worker trainee. For Freud, the tools of transference, dream interpretation, and free association were all designed to achieve the ultimate goal of psychoanalysis: "to make the hidden visible."

Think about this approach to treating mental illness for a moment. If you suffered from depression, obsessions, schizophrenia (like Elena Conway), or panic attacks (like Abigail Abercrombie), then—according to psychoanalytic theory—the best way to relieve your symptoms was to unearth the hidden psychic conflicts generating your pathological behavior. To dig up these conflicts, the psychoanalyst, like the biblical Joseph, might interpret the cryptic significance of your dreams. If you refused to talk about your dreams—if, instead, you wanted to talk about what could be done to prevent you from committing suicide if your depression took hold again—the psychoanalyst would interpret this desire to switch topics as "resistance" that needed to be worked through.

As the popularity of psychoanalysis and the number of its practitioners grew, some of Freud's protégés wanted to push psychoanalysis in new directions and began to propose new ideas about mental illness and the mind that were quite different from Freud's own. Perhaps some psychic conflicts were not linked to sex at all? Might there be a cosmic significance to the unconscious? What about *four* parts to the mind, instead of three?

If Freud was the CEO of the psychoanalytical movement, his management style was more like that of Steve Jobs than of Bill Gates. He wanted complete control of everything, and all designs needed to conform to his own sensibilities. As the society continued to grow and more new ideas were being proposed, the psychoanalytic CEO realized he needed to do something to gain tighter control over the movement and simultaneously bring his ideas to a larger audience. In the language of business, Freud wanted to expand his market share while retaining tight brand control.

He decided to dissolve the increasingly fractious Wednesday Psychological Society—which was still being held in his stuffy, overcrowded parlor—and reconstitute it as a formal professional organization. Only those who were fully committed to Freud's ideas were invited to continue as members; Freud expelled the rest. On April 15, 1908, the new group introduced itself to the public as the Psychoanalytic Society. With just twenty-two members, the fledgling society held the promise of reshaping every inch of psychiatry and captivating the entire world—if it didn't tear itself apart first.

Heretics

Though psychoanalytic theory was catching on and Freud was confident that his daring ideas about mental illness were fundamentally sound, he was quite conscious of the fact that he was on shaky ground with regard to scientific evidence. Rather than reacting to this lack of supporting data by conducting research to fill in the blanks, Freud instead made a decision that would seal the fate of psychoanalysis and critically affect the course of American psychiatry, fossilizing a promising and dynamic scientific theory into a petrified religion.

Freud chose to present his theory in a way that discouraged questioning and thwarted any efforts at verification or falsification. He demanded complete loyalty to his theory, and insisted that his disciples follow his clinical techniques without deviation. As the Psychoanalytic Society grew, the scientist who had once called for skeptical rigor in *A Project for a Scientific Psychology* now presented his hypotheses as articles of faith that must be adhered to with absolute fidelity.

As a psychiatrist who lived through many of the worst excesses of the psychoanalytic theocracy, I regard Freud's fateful decision with sadness and regret. If we are practicing medicine, if we are pursuing science, if we are studying some-thing as vertiginously complicated as the human mind, then we must always be prepared to humbly submit our ideas for replications and verification by others and to modify them as new evidence arises. What was especially disappointing about Freud's insular strategy is that so many core elements of his theory ultimately proved to be accurate, even holding up in the light of contemporary neuroscience research. Freud's the-ory of complementary and competing systems of cognition is basic to modern neuroscience, instantiated in leading neural models of vision, memory, motor control, decision making, and language. The idea, first promulgated by Freud, of pro-gressive stages of mental development forms the cornerstone of the modern fields of developmental psychology and devel-opmental neurobiology. To this day, we don't have a better way of understanding self-defeating, narcissistic, passive-dependent, and passive-aggressive behavior patterns than what Freud proposed.

But along with prescient insights, Freud's theories were also full of missteps, oversights, and outright howlers. We shake our heads now at his conviction that young boys want to marry their mothers and kill their fathers, while a girl's natural sex-ual development drives her to want a penis of her own. As Jus-tice Louis Brandeis so aptly declared, "Sunlight is the best disinfectant," and it seems likely that many of Freud's less cred-ible conjectures would have been scrubbed away by the punc-tilious process of scientific inquiry if they had been treated as testable hypotheses rather than papal edicts.

Instead, anyone who criticized or modified Freud's ideas was considered a blaspheming apostate, denounced as a mor-tal enemy of psychoanalysis, and excommunicated. The most influential founding member of the psychoanalytic movement, Alfred Adler, the man Freud once admiringly called "the only personality there," was the first major figure to be expelled.

Prior to meeting Freud, Adler had already laid out his own views on therapy, emphasizing the need to perceive the patient as a whole person and understand his whole story. In contrast to Freud's theory of a divided consciousness, Adler believed the mind to be indivisible—an *Individuum*. Freud's insistence on interpreting all of a patient's conflicts as sexual in nature, no matter how improbable and far-fetched, also bothered Adler, since he felt that aggression was just as potent a source of psychic conflict.

But there may have been other reasons for their schism. When asked about acrimony among psychiatrists with an obvious reference to the members of the Wednesday Society, Freud replied, "It is not the scientific differences that are so important, it is usually some other kind of animosity, jealousy, or revenge, that gives the impulse to enmity. The scientific differences come later." Freud was aloof, cold, with a laser-focused mind better suited for research than politics. Most of his patients were well-educated members of the upper strata of Viennese society, while the convivial Adler had greater affinity for the working class.

Like Stalin declaring Trotsky persona non grata, in 1911 Freud publicly declared Adler's ideas contrary to the movement and issued an ultimatum to all members of the Psychoanalytic Society to drop Adler or face expulsion themselves. Freud accused Adler of having paranoid delusions and using "terrorist tactics" to undermine the psychoanalytic movement. He whispered to his friends that the revolt by Adler was that of "an abnormal individual driven mad by ambition."

For his own part, Adler's enmity toward Freud endured for the rest of his life. Whenever someone pointed out that he had been an early disciple of Freud, Adler would angrily whip out a time-faded postcard—his invitation to Freud's first coffee klatch—as proof that Freud had initially sought his intellectual companionship, not the other way around. Not long before his death, in 1937, Adler was having dinner in a New York restaurant with the young Abraham Maslow, a psychologist who eventually achieved his own acclaim for the concept of self-actualization. Maslow casually asked Adler about his friendship with Freud. Adler exploded and proceeded to denounce Freud as a swindler and schemer.

Other exiles and defections followed, including that of Wilhelm Stekel, the man who originally came up with the idea for the Wednesday Psychological Society, and Otto Rank, whom Freud for years had called his "loyal helper and co-worker." But the unkindest cut of all, in Freud's eyes, undoubtedly came from the Swiss physician Carl Gustav Jung, his own Brutus.

In 1906, after reading Jung's psychoanalysis-influenced book *Studies in Word-Association*, Freud eagerly invited him to his home in Vienna. The two men, nineteen years apart, immediately recognized each other as kindred spirits. They talked for thirteen hours straight, history not recording whether they paused for food or bathroom breaks. Shortly thereafter, Freud sent a collection of his latest published essays to Jung in Zurich, marking the beginning of an intense correspondence and collaboration that lasted six years. Jung was elected the first president of the International Psychoanalytical Association with Freud's enthusiastic support, and Freud eventually anointed Jung as "his adopted eldest son, his crown prince and successor." But—as with Freud and Adler—the seeds of discord were present in their relationship from the very start.

Jung was deeply spiritual, and his ideas veered toward the mystical. He believed in synchronicity, the idea that apparent coincidences in life—such as the sun streaming through the clouds as you emerge from church after your wedding—were cosmically orchestrated. Jung downplayed the importance of sexual conflicts and instead focused on the quasi-numinous role of the *collective unconscious*—a part of the unconscious, according to Jung, that contains memories and ideas that belong to our entire species.

Freud, in sharp contrast, was an atheist and didn't believe that spirituality or the occult should be connected with psychoanalysis in any way. He claimed to have never experienced any "religious feelings," let alone the mystical feelings that Jung professed. And of course, in Freud's eyes, sexual conflict was the sina qua non of psychoanalysis.

Freud became increasingly concerned that Jung's endorsement of unscientific ideas would harm the movement (ironic, as there were no plans to develop scientific support for Freud's ideas either). Finally, in November of 1912, Jung and Freud met for the last time at a gathering of Freud's inner circle in Munich. Over lunch, the group was discussing a recent psychoanalytic paper about the ancient Egyptian pharaoh Amenhotep. Jung commented that too much had been made of the fact that Amenhotep had ordered his father's name erased from all inscriptions. Freud took this personally, denouncing Jung for leaving Freud's name off his recent publications, working himself into such a frenzy that he fell to the floor in a dead faint. Not long after, the two colleagues parted ways for good, Jung abandoning psychoanalytic theory entirely for his own form of psychiatry, which he called, with an obvious debt to Freud, "analytical psychology."

Despite the tensions within the fracturing psychoanalytic movement, by 1910 psychoanalysis had become the *traitement du jour* in continental Europe and established itself as one of the most popular forms of therapy among the upper and middle classes, especially among affluent Jews. Psychoanalytic theory also became highly influential in the arts, shaping the work of novelists, painters, and playwrights. But although by 1920 every educated European had heard of Freud, psychoanalysis never wholly dominated European psychiatry. Even at its high-water mark in Europe, psychoanalysis competed with several

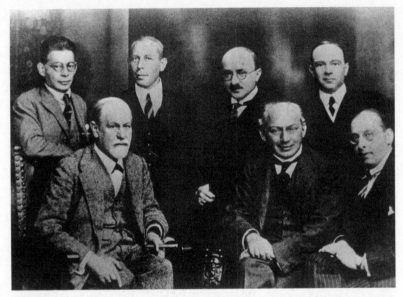

Sigmund Freud's inner circle of the Psychoanalytic Society. From left to right are Otto Rank, Freud, Karl Abraham, Max Eitingon, Sándor Ferenczi, Ernest Jones, Hanns Sachs. (HIP/Art Resource, NY)

other approaches to mental illness, including Gestalt theory, phenomenological psychiatry, and social psychiatry, while in the United States, psychoanalysis failed to gain any traction at all.

Then, in the late 1930s, a sudden twist of history obliterated psychoanalysis from the face of continental Europe. After the rise of the Nazis, Freud and his theory would never regain their standing on the Continent they had enjoyed in the early decades of the twentieth century. At the same time, the chain of events initiated by German fascism roused psychoanalysis from its American slumber and invigorated a new Freudian force in North America that would systematically take over every institution of American psychiatry—and soon beget the shrink.

A Plague upon America

While nineteenth-century European psychiatry oscillated like a metronome between psychodynamic and biological theories, before the arrival of Freud there was precious little that could be mistaken for progress in American psychiatry. American medicine had benefited, by varying degrees, from advances in surgery, vaccines, antiseptic principles, nursing, and germ theory coming from European medical schools, but the medicine of mental health remained in hibernation.

The origins of American psychiatry are traditionally traced to Benjamin Rush, one of the signers of the Declaration of Independence. He is considered a Founding Father of the United States, and through the sepia mists of time he has acquired another paternal appellation: Father of American Psychiatry. Rush was considered the "New World" Pinel for advocating that mental illness and addictions were medical illnesses, not moral failings, and for unshackling the inmates of the Pennsylvania Hospital in 1780.

However, while Rush did publish the first textbook on mental illness in the United States, the 1812 tome *Medical Inquiries and Observations upon the Diseases of the Mind,* he did not encourage or pursue experimentation and evidence-gathering to support his thesis and organized his descriptions of mental illness around theories he found personally compelling. Rush believed, for instance, that many mental illnesses were caused by the disruption of blood circulation. (It is interesting to observe that before the advent of modern neuroscience so many psychiatrists envisioned mental illness as some variant of a clogged sewage pipe, with disorders arising from the obstructed flow of some essential biological medium: Mesmer's magnetic channels, Reich's orgone energy, Rush's blood circulation.)

To improve circulation to the mentally ill brain, Rush treated patients with a special device of his own invention: the Rotational Chair. The base of the chair was connected to an iron axle that could be rotated rapidly by means of a hand crank. A psychotic patient would be strapped snugly into the chair and then spun around and around like an amusement park Tilt-A-Whirl until his psychotic symptoms were blotted out by dizziness, disorientation, and vomiting.

Rush believed that another source of mental illness was sensory overload. Too much visual and auditory stimulation, he claimed, unhinged the mind. To combat excessive mental input, he invented the Tranquilizer Chair. First, a patient was strapped to a sturdy chair. Next, a wooden box that vaguely resembled a birdhouse was lowered over his head, depriving him of sight and sound and rendering sneezing a very awkward affair.

But Rush's preferred method for treating insanity was more straightforward: purging the bowels. He fabricated his own customized "Bilious Pills" filled with "10 grains of calomel and 15 grains of jalap"—powerful laxatives made from mercury, the poisonous quicksilver found in old thermometers. His patients endowed the pills with a more colorful moniker: "Rush's thunderbolts." Opening up the bowels, Rush attested, expelled any deleterious substances causing mental illness, along with the previous day's breakfast, lunch, and dinner. Unfortunately, modern science has yet to uncover any evidence that mental illness can be cured through defecation.

Rush recognized that the very individuals whom he regarded as most in need of his gut-clearing remedies—the manic and psychotic—often actively resisted the good doctor's medicine. Undeterred, he devised a solution. "It is sometimes difficult to prevail upon patients in this state of madness to take mercury in any of the ways in which it is usually administered," he wrote. "In these cases I have succeeded by sprinkling a few grains of

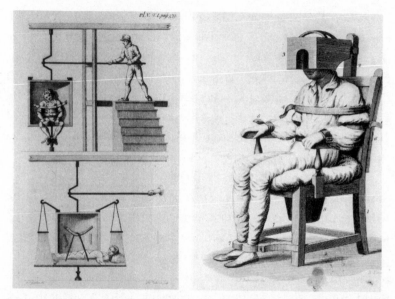

Rotational Chair and Tranquilizer Chair, nineteenth-century treatment for mental illness in the U.S. (U.S. National Library of Medicine)

calomel daily upon a piece of bread, and afterwards spreading over it a thin covering of butter." Between the nauseating spinning chairs and the constant evacuation of bowels, one guesses that a psychiatric ward in Rush's hospital could be a very messy place.

Rush's medical celebrity came less from his Rube Goldberg–like treatments than from his policies and advocacy for the mentally ill. After seeing the appalling conditions of mental patients in Philadelphia's Pennsylvania Hospital, Rush led a successful campaign in 1792 for the state to build a separate mental ward where the patients could be housed more compassionately. And while Rush's thunderbolts and whirligigs might seem misguided and even a bit harebrained, they were certainly more humane than the beatings and chains that were the norm in asylums at the turn of the eighteenth century.

When Freud arrived in New York in 1909, American psychiatry was firmly established as a profession of alienists toiling in mental asylums. There was precious little originality in psychiatric research, which consisted of uninspired papers with titles like "The Imbecile with Criminal Instincts" and "The Effects of Exercise upon the Retardation of Conditions of Depression." In an intellectual landscape as dry and barren as this was, any new spark might set off a conflagration.

Freud's first and only visit to the United States occurred in September of 1909, shortly before World War I. He crossed the Atlantic on the ocean liner *George Washington* with Carl Jung, with whom he was still on intimate terms. It was the height of psychoanalytic unity, just before Freud's acolytes started splintering off, and Freud believed that his novel ideas about the mind might shake American psychiatry from its lethargy. When the ship docked in New York, he reportedly said to Jung, "They don't realize that we are bringing them the plague." Freud's comment would eventually seem more prescient than he realized.

Freud had come to the States at the request of G. Stanley Hall, the first American to receive a doctorate in psychology and the founder of the American Psychological Association. Hall had invited Freud to receive an honorary doctorate from Clark University, in Worcester, Massachusetts, where Hall was president, and to give a series of public lectures. These talks marked the first public recognition of Freud's work in the United States.

It is interesting to note that it was psychologists who expressed the interest and took the initiative to invite Freud and expose America to his ideas. Psychology (translated as "study of the soul") was a fledgling discipline that the German physician Wilhelm Wundt is credited with founding in 1879. Wundt was trained in anatomy and physiology, but when the anatomical study of mental functions led to a dead end, he turned to the outward manifestations of the brain reflected in human behavior and established an experimental laboratory devoted to behavior at the University of Leipzig.

William James, also a physician, almost contemporaneously became the leading proponent and scholar on psychology in the United States. Like Wundt, James was a devoted empiricist who believed in the value of evidence and experimentation. It is notable that the lack of a path forward in the traditional research paradigms of medical research led psychiatrically minded physicians to invoke psychology as their scientific discipline. Hence the invitation to Freud.

It is interesting to note that the discipline of psychology stems from physicians whose work, in the late nineteenth and early twentieth centuries, to understand mental functions using (then) traditional methods of medical research had been thwarted and who were compelled to pursue their goals by unconventional means. It is also notable that the early pioneers of psychology (Wundt, James, Hermann von Ebbinghaus, and subsequently Ivan Pavlov and then B. F. Skinner) were ardent empiricists devoted to research. And while Freud was similarly driven to develop psychological constructs to explain mental functions and illnesses by the same obstacles, he eschewed systematic research or any form of empirical validation of his theory.

At the time of his visit, Freud was virtually unknown in America; he wasn't even the headliner when Clark sent out notices of his talk. There was no media coverage of Freud's arrival before his talk and precious little afterward, apart from *The Nation*'s coverage of the event: "One of the most attractive of the eminent foreign savants who came was Sigmund Freud of Vienna. Far too little is known in America of either the man or his work. His views are now beginning to be talked of in Germany as the psychology of the future, as Wagner's music was once dubbed the music of the future."

Freud was an articulate and persuasive speaker who rarely failed to impress educated men and women. In both Europe and America, some of the greatest scientific and medical minds met with him and almost all came away converted. Attendees at Freud's talks at Clark included James, who was so impressed by Freud that he said, "The future of psychology belongs to your work."

Another attendee, the anarchist Emma Goldman, known for founding *Mother Earth* magazine, distributing birth control, and trying to assassinate the chairman of Carnegie Steel, was also smitten. "Only people of depraved minds," she later claimed, "could impugn the motives or find 'impure' so great and fine a personality as Freud." The great and fine personality of Freud was invited by James Jackson Putnam, the highly influential professor of nervous system diseases at Harvard, to visit him at his country retreat. After four days of intensive discussion, Putnam embraced Freud's theory and publicly endorsed the man and his work. Not long afterward, Putnam co-organized the first meeting of the American Psychoanalytic Association (APsaA), which would quickly become the most influential psychoanalytic organization in the United States, not that there was much competition.

Despite the warm reception and lavish kudos, Freud's impact on American psychiatry was initially quite modest. Two decades later, the American Psychoanalytic Association had still only attracted ninety-two members nationwide. Though psychoanalysis had begun to catch on among wealthy and educated patients in New York City suffering from mild disorders—duplicating Freud's earlier success in the cosmopolitan city of Vienna—it did not penetrate into universities and medical schools, and failed to make any dent whatsoever in asylum psychiatry, still the hegemonic force in American mental health care.

In 1930, if you had told a psychiatrist that Freudian psychoanalysis would soon dominate American psychiatry, he would have considered that preposterous. There was little reason to believe that psychoanalysis would ever spread outside of a few cities on the East Coast. But then Hitler's rise to power and aggression abruptly brought Europe to the brink of war, destabilizing the governments and boundaries of countries. It had a similar effect on the state and boundaries of psychiatry. While fascism spelled the end of psychoanalysis in Europe, it launched the unexpected rise of a psychoanalytic empire in America.

In the late nineteenth and early twentieth century, anti-Semitism was disturbingly common in Europe. Though Freud was an avowed atheist, he was ethnically Jewish, and he feared that if psychoanalysis developed a Jewish association in the public mind it would be doomed. From the start he worked hard to downplay any potential connection between psychoanalytic ideas and Jewishness. This was one of the reasons—probably the main reason—that Freud pushed for Carl Jung to become the first president of the International Psychoanalytical Association. Jung, who was Swiss, was neither Viennese nor Jewish, and his presidency would send a strong public signal that psychoanalysis was not a Jewish cabal. Nevertheless, Freud's advocacy for Jung drew angry protests from Adler and Stekel. Freud's oldest supporters felt that a member of the original Viennese group should be given the post. When Adler and Stekel confronted Freud, Freud declared that he needed the support of another country (Switzerland) to counter the perceived anti-Semitic hostility surrounding them in Vienna, dramatically pulling off his coat and shouting: "My enemies would be willing to see me starve; they would tear my very coat off my back!"

But despite Freud's best efforts, psychoanalysis was inextricably linked to Jewish culture. Freud's inner circle was almost entirely Jewish, as were the vast majority of the first generation of psychoanalysts, and they tended to believe that being Jewish helped one appreciate Freud's wisdom. Many early psychoanalytic patients were drawn from affluent Jewish communities. At the peak of the Wednesday Psychological Society, the only non-Jewish member was Ernest Jones, an English neurologist from London. Sándor Ferenczi, a close confidant of Freud and an early president of the International Psychoanalytical Association, remarked about Jones's lonely presence: "It has seldom been so clear to me as now what a psychological advantage it signifies to be born a Jew." According to historian Edward Shorter, the subtext of much of the early psychoanalytic movement was: "We Jews have given a precious gift to modern civilization."

As Hitler's Nazism strengthened its hold on central Europe — especially in Austria, the capital of psychoanalysis — many psychoanalysts fled to safer countries. Shortly after Hitler's ascent to power, there was a bonfire of psychoanalytic books in the center of Berlin, including all of Freud's. Dr. M. H. Göring (cousin of Hermann Göring, Hitler's second-in-command) took over the German Society for Psychotherapy, the leading psychiatric organization in Germany, and purged it of all Jewish and psychoanalytic elements, remaking it into the Reich Institute for Psychological Research and Psychotherapy.

Freud stayed in Vienna as long as he could, even enduring a swastika flag draped across his building's doorway, until one spring day in 1938 Nazi soldiers raided his second-floor apartment. His wife, Martha, asked them to leave their rifles in the hall. The commander stiffly addressed the master of the house as "Herr Professor" and bid his men to search the entire apartment for contraband. Once the soldiers had finally left, Martha Freud informed her husband that they had seized about $840 in Austrian shillings. "Dear me," the eighty-two-year-old Freud remarked, "I have never taken that much for a single visit."

But Freud would end up paying even more to the Nazis for an exit visa that would allow him to take both his family and possessions to Britain: about $200,000 in contemporary currency. The money for the "exit tax" was raised by sales of Freud's papers and artifacts and by the generous contribution of an admirer of Freud named Marie Bonaparte; the entire exit operation was surreptitiously facilitated by the Nazi "commissar" who directed the raid on Freud's home. (Another Jewish refugee fled Vienna with his family around the same time but with much less notoriety: nine-year-old Eric Kandel, who would be inspired by Freud to become a psychiatrist and go on to win the Nobel Prize for brain research.) Practically overnight, the movement launched by Freud was snuffed out in Europe.

Although Freud himself immigrated to London, most psychoanalyst émigrés sought refuge in America, particularly in the big cities and especially New York. For those in the movement, it was as if the Vatican and its cardinals had shifted the site of the Holy See from Rome to Manhattan. Having been analyzed or trained directly by the master himself, these émigrés were welcomed as royalty by the fledgling psychoanalytic movement in the United States. They were granted professorships in leading universities, wrote popular books, and established psychoanalytic institutes.

These psychiatric refugees would soon change the fundamental nature of mental health care in the United States, but not necessarily for the better. They brought with them the dogmatic and faith-based approach to psychiatry that Freud had espoused, discouraging inquiry and experimentation. Eventually, just as Freud predicted, psychoanalysis would become a plague upon American medicine, infecting every institution of psychiatry with its dogmatic and antiscientific mind-set. But this resistance to research and empirical verification was only part of the problem.

All of the immigrant psychoanalytic luminaries were displaced Jews, fleeing persecution. They had been trained by Jews, had mostly Jewish patients, and had undergone harrowing experiences as refugees from a brutally anti-Semitic regime. By 1940, American psychoanalysis had become a unique phenomenon in the annals of medicine: a scientifically ungrounded theory, adapted for the specific psychic needs of a minority ethnic group. It would be hard to imagine a therapy less suited to the treatment of people with severe mental illness.

The Rise of the Shrink

The American Psychiatric Association (APA) is the premier professional organization for psychiatrists in the United States and is best known to the public as the publisher of the *Diagnostic and Statistical Manual of Mental Illness*. The APA is also the oldest active medical organization in America, founded in 1844 as the Association of Medical Superintendents of American Institutions for the Insane. (By comparison, the American Medical Association was founded in 1847.)

For the first century of its existence, the APA was almost exclusively a society of alienists. In 1890, the APA adopted the image of Benjamin Rush for its seal, and Rush's face remains on the official APA emblem to this day. By the time Freud visited the States in 1909, the APA had changed its name to the American Medico-Psychological Association (reflecting the emphasis on psychology that Freud had orchestrated and Wundt and James had embraced) even though its members still mostly worked in institutions for the insane, and they remained alienists in 1921 when they adopted the organization's present appellation.

In the first couple of decades after Freud's visit to the United States, the members of the APA weren't particularly interested in his unsubstantiated theories about unconscious conflicts, which appeared to have little relevance for the screaming and suicidal inmates of overcrowded asylums. On the other hand, American psychoanalysts most certainly cared about the APA. Beginning in 1924, the American Psychoanalytic Association held their meetings at the same time and in the same city as the much larger American Psychiatric Association. In the early 1930s, the APsaA began pushing hard for the APA to officially recognize the psychoanalytic approach to psychiatry, igniting a portentous conflict within the executive board of the APA.

At first, the leading alienists of the APA resisted endorsing Freud's theories, which they termed unscientific and unproven. Eventually, though, the mood began to shift, as the alienists came to realize that, science aside, psychoanalysis offered a distinct benefit for their profession: a way out of the asylum. For almost a century, the most prominent role a psychiatrist could hope to obtain in the medical field was to be a director of an asylum, an alienist in a country madhouse overseeing a horde of incurables, working apart from one's medical colleagues, separated from mainstream society. In contrast, neurologists had by this time developed pleasant and lucrative office practices outside of hospitals, where they could obtain generous fees from well-heeled patients for tending to headaches, muscle paralysis, and fainting, among other maladies. Neurologists looked down their noses at their country bumpkin psychiatric cousins, and even the most eminent of alienists resented their lowly status. The psychiatrist Frank Braceland, who often presided over meetings of psychiatrists and neurologists when he served as the director of the American Board of Psychiatry and Neurology from 1946 to 1952, described the relations of the sibling professions in the 1940s to me when I interviewed him for a historical documentary film in 1979:

> It was impossible to get neurologists and psychiatrists to sit down together, because neither side liked one another much. The neurologists thought that neurology was the "Queen of Medicine" and psychiatry was the jester. The psychiatrists, meanwhile, insisted the neurologists preached neurology but practiced psychiatry.

Now, for the first time in psychiatry's inglorious history, Freud's remarkable new therapy of psychoanalysis granted alienists the opportunity to establish office-based practices of their own. Whether a devotee of Freud, Adler, Jung, or Rank, the psychoanalyst could treat wealthy patients with minor mental maladies in the civil environs of a comfortably appointed drawing room.

Of course, embracing psychoanalysis meant embracing a radical redefinition of mental illness. Previously, the boundary between sick and healthy was drawn between those who *needed* to be institutionalized and those who *did not* need to be institutionalized. To be mentally ill meant one was *seriously* mentally ill—suffering from unhinged psychosis, debilitating depression, heedless mania, or a sizable diminution of intellect. But Freud blurred the boundary between mental illness and mental health, since psychoanalytic theory suggested that almost everyone had some kind of neurotic conflict that could be resolved with proper (psychoanalytic) treatment. Psychoanalysis introduced a new type of psychiatric patient, a person who could function effectively in society but who wanted to function even better. Today, these types of patients are known as the *worried well*.

The worried well became the primary market for psychoanalysis in both Europe and the United States, fueling its ascent. In 1917, only about 8 percent of American psychiatrists were in private practice. By 1941, this figure had increased to 38 percent, largely because of the adoption of psychoanalysis. By the 1960s, more than 66 percent of all American psychiatrists were in private practice. Instead of wearing white coats and shouldering through a daily grind of raving and catatonic inmates, psychiatrists could chat with well-heeled businessmen about their childhood memories and gently guide well-coiffed matrons through their free-associations.

Even better, psychoanalysis bestowed on psychiatrists a

meaningful and active role in treatment: Like omen-divining wizards, they interpreted the private emotional experiences of their patients and drew upon their intellect and creativity to formulate elaborate diagnoses and orchestrate complex treatments. Instead of hapless caretakers for the insane, they became *consiglieri* for the wealthy, educated, and influential. They were alienists no longer. They had become *shrinks*.

The term "headshrinker" first originated in the 1940s in the offices and backlots of Hollywood and reflected the emerging new role for psychiatrists. During this era, adventure films were the rage in movie palaces, especially movies set in exotic jungles where cannibal tribes often shrank the heads of enemies. Since the name of the person who first applied the term "headshrinkers" to psychiatrists is lost to history, we don't know for certain whether he intended to suggest that psychoanalysts were shrinking the big egos of movie stars down to size or was comparing psychoanalysis to the primeval sorcery of the jungle witch doctor. The latter seems more likely. One of the first appearances of "headshrinker" in print was in a 1948 letter to the editor in the *Baltimore Sun*, penned by a psychoanalyst in response to an article by noted Baltimore writer H. L. Mencken that had lambasted Freudian therapy as "hooey." The psychoanalyst retorted, "Mencken should examine the syllabus of the requirements necessary for certification before damning these gentlemen as witch doctors, head shrinkers, totemists, and voodooists."

It seems appropriate that Hollywood, with its culture of self-absorption, self-improvement, and pretense, was one of the first communities to embrace a new therapy that involved endless self-examination. A 1949 scholarly study of cartoons in popular magazines documented the transition taking place within psychiatry. "Older cartoons about psychiatry portray only psychotic patients in insane asylums," concludes the author. "There is no *psychiatrist* portrayed because psychiatry was not a profession then. The number of cartoons about psychiatrists greatly increased in the 1930s and 1940s until they became even more frequent than cartoons about general practitioners and ministers."

The term "headshrinker" entered broad use after a 1950 *Time* magazine article about Western "B" movie actor Hopalong Cassidy, which stated, "Anyone who had predicted that he would end up as the rootin'-tootin' idol of U.S. children would have been led instantly off to a headshrinker.*" The asterisked footnote read: "Hollywood jargon for a psychiatrist." By the mid-1950s, the entire country was using the term, which made its way into the lyrics of the 1957 Broadway musical *West Side Story*:

> JETS: We're disturbed, we're disturbed,
>   We're the most disturbed,
>   Like we're psychologic'ly disturbed.
> DIESEL: In the opinion of this court, this child is depraved
>   on account he ain't had a normal home.
> ACTION: Hey, I'm depraved on account I'm deprived.
> DIESEL: So take him to a headshrinker.

Emboldened by their growing influence, American psychoanalysts in the 1940s aspired to even greater prominence and power. Knowing that the path to influence ran through medical schools and teaching hospitals, psychoanalysts began targeting universities. A 1940 *Bulletin of the American Psychoanalytic Association* encourages its members to "secure a formal contract from a near-by university," and later asserts that "it is to the interest of psychiatry, and especially to the development of psychoanalytic psychiatry, that our psychoanalytic training institutes should teach more men who are heading towards academic teaching positions in medical schools and towards positions in hospitals." One by one, Case Western Reserve, the

University of Pittsburgh, the University of California at San Francisco, Johns Hopkins, the University of Pennsylvania, Columbia, Stanford, Yale, and Harvard saw analysts ascend to their department chairs, and each new conquest was celebrated as a triumph within the psychoanalytic movement.

By 1960, almost every major psychiatry position in the country was occupied by a psychoanalyst. There were twenty psychoanalytic training institutes across the United States, many affiliated with psychiatry departments at top universities. The American Psychoanalytic Association swelled from 92 members in 1932 (when the first European émigrés began to arrive) to about 1,500 in 1960. By then, virtually all clinical psychiatrists—whether formally credentialed or not—were psychoanalytically oriented. In 1924, the first Freud-leaning psychiatrist was elected president of the APA, and the next fifty-eight years witnessed an almost unbroken series of psychoanalyst presidents of the American Psychiatric Association.

William Menninger, one of the most famous and respected of American psychoanalysts, became the face of American psychiatry and enthusiastically promoted his profession in the media; in 1948, *Time* magazine featured Menninger on its cover, labeling him "psychiatry's U.S. sales manager." He was so influential that he was able to secure a personal meeting with President Harry Truman in 1948 and prevailed upon him to send "a message of greeting" to the joint meeting of the APA and APsaA. Truman wrote: "Never have we had a more pressing need for experts in human engineering. The greatest prerequisite for peace must be sanity, which permits clear thinking on the part of all citizens. We must continue to look to experts in the field of psychiatry and other mental sciences for guidance." By "psychiatry and mental sciences," the president meant psychoanalysis. By "experts in human engineering," he meant shrinks.

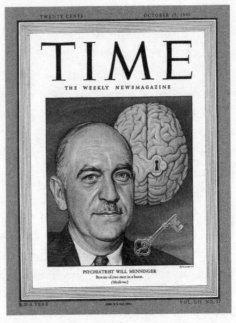

William Menninger on the cover of *Time* magazine. (*Time*, October 25, 1948, © Time, Inc. Used under license)

Schizophrenogenic Mothers and World Peace

From their positions of influence in university medical schools and the APA, psychoanalysts could now dictate the training of future psychiatrists. Curricula based upon biological and behavioral theories were minimized, while Freud-influenced ideas became the core of virtually every medical school program in psychiatry—and, indeed, became an all-embracing worldview that permeated the training of every aspiring psychiatrist. In addition to attending lectures on psychoanalysis and having their cases supervised by analysts, if a medical student wanted to be a psychiatrist she had to undergo a "successful" psychoanalysis herself during postgraduate training.

Think about that for a minute. The only way to become a

psychiatrist—a bona fide medical professional—was to share your life's history, innermost feelings, fears, and aspirations, your nightly dreams and daily fantasies, with someone who would use this deeply intimate material to determine how devoted you were to Freudian principles. Imagine if the only way you could become a theoretical physicist was to confess an unwavering and unquestioning dedication to the theory of relativity or the precepts of quantum mechanics, or if the only way you could become an economist was to reveal whether Karl Marx appeared as an angel (or devil) in your dreams. If a trainee wanted to rise within the ranks of academic psychiatry or develop a successful practice, she had to demonstrate fealty to psychoanalytic theory. If not, she risked being banished to working in the public-hospital sector, which usually meant a state mental institution. If you were looking for an indoctrination method to foster a particular ideology within a profession, you probably couldn't do much better than forcing all job applicants to undergo confessional psychotherapy with a therapist-inquisitor already committed to the ideology.

If an established psychiatrist who had somehow been trained outside of the Freudian paradigm questioned the validity of psychoanalysis, he was shouted down at conferences and/or branded with a diagnosis such as passive-aggressive personality disorder or narcissistic personality disorder or termed a sociopath. In 1962, the influential psychiatrist Leon Eisenberg offered a few critical remarks about the unscientific nature of psychoanalysis at a medical educators' meeting. "There was a veritable stampede of Department Chairmen to the floor microphones. Just about every eminent figure present rose to defend the primacy of psychoanalysis as 'the basic science' of psychiatry," lamented Eisenberg, according to Hannah Decker's excellent book *The Making of DSM-III*.

Under the psychoanalytic hegemony, psychiatrists in training were discouraged from bothering with the kinds of patients who usually ended up in asylums and mental institutions, patients like Elena Conway, in preference of treating patients with milder ailments and more amenable to psychoanalysis. The treatment of the seriously mentally ill—psychiatry's original and primary mandate—was subordinated to the treatment of the worried well. Edward Shorter's *A History of Psychiatry* shares the recollections of a psychiatry resident at the Delaware State Hospital in the 1940s:

> It was urgently driven home that we should view institutional psychiatry merely as a brief transitional stage for us. Our ideal professional goal was doing psychoanalysis in private practice in combination with supervising training at one of the psychoanalytic institutes independent of a university department. From the viewpoint of the psychoanalytic theories of the 1940s, our daily therapeutic activities at Delaware Hospital were considered highly questionable. The somatic therapies, so we were told, were stopgaps. They concealed instead of uncovering. Ordering a sedative for an agitated psychotic patient was not therapeutic for the patient but instead considered an anxiety reaction on the part of the doctor.

Having conquered academic psychiatry and created an industry of private practice for this specialty, American psychoanalysts reevaluated the potency of their therapeutic métier and now concluded it was even stronger medicine than originally believed. Freud himself had declared that psychoanalysis was not easily applied to schizophrenia and manic-depressive illness, and the master's words had prompted the majority of psychoanalysts to avoid treating patients with severe mental illness. But as the twentieth century progressed, American psychoanalysts began to assert that it *was* possible to convince the schizophrenics to give up their delusions, coax the manics out of their mania, and cajole the autistics away from their autism. The American psychoanalytical movement launched a new initiative: turning alienists into analysts.

One of the progenitors of this professional transmutation was the Swiss-educated psychiatrist Adolf Meyer, who immigrated in 1892 to the U.S., where he initially practiced neurology and neuropathology. In 1902, he became director of the New York State Pathological Institute (now called the New York State Psychiatric Institute), where he began to argue that severe mental illness resulted from personality dysfunction rather than brain pathology—and that Freud's theories offered the best explanation of how these personality dysfunctions led to illness. In 1913, Meyer became chair of the first psychiatric inpatient clinic in a general hospital in the U.S., at Johns Hopkins University, and began to apply the newly arrived psychoanalytic methods to the clinic's schizophrenic and manic-depressive patients.

Influenced by Meyer's pioneering work in Baltimore, two nearby institutions in Maryland became flagship hospitals for using psychoanalysis to treat the severely mentally ill: the Chestnut Lodge Sanitarium and the Sheppard and Enoch Pratt Hospital. In 1922, psychiatrist Harry Stack Sullivan arrived at Sheppard Pratt. In Sullivan's view, schizophrenia was the result of "anxiety reactions"—the unsuccessful adjustment to life's stresses—and only occurred in individuals who failed to have satisfying sexual experiences. Under the mentorship of Adolf Meyer, Sullivan developed one of the earliest psychoanalytic methods for treating schizophrenic patients. Since he believed that schizophrenics were having difficulty integrating their life experiences into a coherent personal narrative, he sought out hospital staff members with personal backgrounds similar to each schizophrenic patient and encouraged these staff to engage in informal conversation with the patient in hopes of providing meaning and coherence to the schizophrenic's "masses of life experience."

Soon, other psychoanalytic hospitals opened around the country. Along with Chestnut Lodge and Sheppard Pratt, McLean Hospital near Boston, Austen Riggs in Stockbridge, Massachusetts, and the Bloomingdale Insane Asylum in New York City became bastions of psychoanalytic treatment for the severely mentally ill—for those who could afford it. It was the Menninger Clinic in Topeka, Kansas, that most famously exemplified the marriage of psychoanalysis and asylum psychiatry. Operated by three generations of the Menninger family, the clinic was a self-contained compound in a pristine rural location (as had been described by Johann Reil over a century earlier) patronized by affluent patients who remained for long periods of time—sometimes years—while undergoing free association, dream analysis, and the other ingredients of intensive psychoanalysis. The Menninger Clinic became the leading American institution for psychiatric treatment for about five decades; during that time, trekking to Topeka was the psychiatric equivalent of a miracle-seeking invalid's journey to a holy shrine. (Woody Allen joked ruefully about the unending duration of analytic therapy and slow pace of results, "I'm going to give my analyst one more year and then I am going to Lourdes.") Among the celebrities who availed themselves of the clinic's revitalizing services were Dorothy Dandridge, Judy Garland, Robert Walker, Marilyn Monroe, and, more recently, Brett Favre.

Mental illnesses that had eluded explanation for one and a half centuries—defying alienists, biological psychiatrists, and psychodynamic psychiatrists alike—now became the subject of a new form of post-Freudian psychoanalytic interpretation. In 1935, Frieda Fromm-Reichmann, a psychoanalyst émigré from Germany (best known as the fictionalized psychiatrist in

I Never Promised You a Rose Garden), arrived at Chestnut Lodge, where she set about revising Sullivan's ideas about schizophrenia. In Fromm-Reichmann's view, schizophrenia was not caused by anxiety reactions in the patient; it was induced by the patient's mother. "The schizophrenic is painfully distrustful and resentful of other people," she wrote, "due to the severe early smothering and rejection he encountered in important people of his infancy and childhood—as a rule, mainly in a 'schizophrenogenic' mother."

According to Fromm-Reichmann, a schizophrenogenic mother provoked psychosis in her child through a toxic pattern of behavior. Naturally, this formulation did not come as welcome news to the parents of schizophrenic children. But not to worry, Fromm-Reichmann assured them; since schizophrenia reflected buried psychological conflicts placed there by the parents, it could be treated with an extended course of talk therapy.

After Fromm-Reichmann, the parents—and particularly the mother—became the appointed source of all varieties of mental illness: Since a person's early psychosexual development was the soil from which all illness grew, psychoanalysis declared that Mom and Dad were the prime candidates for psychopathic culpability. The prominent anthropologist Gregory Bateson, husband of Margaret Mead and a researcher at the Mental Research Institute in California, postulated a "double bind" theory of schizophrenia, which appointed the mother as the sickest member of the family. According to Bateson, mothers fostered schizophrenia in their children by issuing conflicting demands (the double bind)—for example, by simultaneously insisting, "Speak when you are spoken to!" and "Don't talk back!" or telling a child to "take initiatives and do something" and then criticizing her for doing something without permission. He argued that the ego resolved this no-win situation by retreating into a fantasy world where the impossible became possible—where, for example, turtles could fly and one could simultaneously speak and be silent.

Autism? Engendered by the "refrigerator mother"—a caregiver who was cold and emotionless toward her children. Homosexuality? Induced by domineering mothers who instilled a fear of castration in their sons along with a deep-seated rejection of women. Depression? "The ego tries to punish itself to forestall punishment by the parent," declared the eminent psychoanalyst Sándor Radó. In other words, suicidal thoughts were the result of your childhood anger toward Mom and Dad getting turned inward onto yourself, since you couldn't express your true feelings to your parents without fearing their reprisal. Paranoia? "It arises in the first six months of life," pronounced analyst Melanie Klein, "as the child spits out the mother's milk, fearing the mother will revenge herself because of his hatred of her."

It was not enough that parents had to endure the tragedy of a child's mental illness; after this onslaught of inane diagnostic formulations, they also had to suffer the indignity of being blamed for the illness because of their own misbehavior. Still worse were the prescribed treatments. Schizophrenia and bipolar disorder—illnesses that for centuries were so mystifying that the only effective treatment was institutionalization—were now believed to be curable through the right kind of talk therapy. Like a pet cat in a tree, a deranged individual merely had to be coaxed into climbing down to reality. This belief led to situations that ranged from the ridiculous (a psychiatrist urging a psychotic person to talk about his sexual fantasies) to the disastrous (a psychiatrist encouraging a suicidal patient to accept that her parents never loved her). As someone who has worked with thousands of schizophrenic patients, I can assure you that they are just as likely to be talked out of their illness as they are to be bled or purged out of it.

By 1955, a majority of psychoanalysts had concluded that *all* forms of mental illness—including neuroses and psychoses—were manifestations of inner psychological conflicts. But the hubris of the American psychoanalytic movement didn't stop there. At this point, if it had been able to lie upon its own therapeutic couch, the psychoanalytic movement would have been diagnosed with all the classic symptoms of mania: extravagant behaviors, grandiose beliefs, and irrational faith in its world-changing powers.

Having folded the seriously mentally ill into their expanding diagnostic tent, psychoanalysts now wanted to include the rest of the human race under their circus Big Top. "Gone forever is the notion that the mentally ill person is an exception," wrote Karl Menninger (William's older brother), in his 1963 bestseller, *The Vital Balance.* "It is now accepted that most people have some degree of mental illness at some time." The book gave detailed advice to readers on how to cope with the stresses of "everyday human life" and "mental disorganization." By embracing psychoanalysis, Menninger declared, it was possible to achieve "a state of being weller than well." Thus did psychoanalysis cross over from a medical profession into a human potential movement.

It was no longer acceptable to divide human behavior into normal and pathological, since virtually all human behavior reflected some form of neurotic conflict, and while conflict was innate to everyone, like fingerprints and belly buttons, no two conflicts looked exactly alike. Starting in the late 1950s and early '60s, the psychoanalysts set out to convince the public that we were *all* walking wounded, normal neurotics, functioning psychotics...and that Freud's teachings contained the secrets to eradicating inner strife and reaching our full potential as human beings.

Yet even this aspirational decree was still not sufficient for the ambition of the psychoanalysts. The movement believed that Freud's theory was so profound that it could solve the political and social problems of the time. A group of psycho-analysts led by William Menninger formed the Group for the Advancement of Psychiatry (GAP), which in 1950 issued a report entitled "The Social Responsibility of Psychiatry: A Statement of Orientation," advocating social activism against war, poverty, and racism. Although these goals were laudable, psychiatry's faith in its power to achieve them was quixotic. Nevertheless, the report helped persuade the APA to shift its focus toward the resolution of significant social problems and even helped shape the agenda of the largest federal institution devoted to mental illness research.

On April 15, 1949, Harry Truman formally established the National Institute of Mental Health (NIMH) and appointed Robert Felix, a practicing psychoanalyst, as its first director. In the psychoanalytically decreed spirit of social activism, Felix announced that early psychiatric intervention in a community setting using psychoanalysis could prevent mild mental ill-nesses from becoming incurable psychoses. Felix explicitly for-bade NIMH expenditures on mental institutions and refused to fund biological research, including research on the brain, since he believed that the future of psychiatry lay in commu-nity activism and social engineering. The energetic and charis-matic Felix was adept at organizational politics, and persuaded Congress and philanthropic agencies that mental illness could only be prevented if the stressors of racism, poverty, and igno-rance were eliminated. From 1949 to 1964, the message com-ing out of the largest research institution in American psychiatry was *not:* "We will find answers to mental illness in the brain." The message was: "If we improve society, then we can eradicate mental illness."

Inspired by the urgings of GAP and NIMH, psychoanalysts pressured their professional organizations to take a stand against U.S. involvement in Vietnam and school segregation; they "marched with Martin Luther King on psychiatric grounds." The psychoanalysts didn't just want to save your soul; they wanted to save the world.

By the 1960s, the psychoanalytic movement had assumed the trappings of a religion. Its leading practitioners suggested that we were all neurotic sinners, but that repentance and forgiveness could be found on the psychoanalytical couch. The words of Jesus might have been attributed to Freud himself: "I am the way, and the truth, and the life; no one comes to the Father but through Me." Psychoanalysts were consulted by government agencies and Congress, were profiled by *Time* and *Life,* and became frequent guests on talk shows. Being "shrunk" had become the ne plus ultra of upper-middle-class American life.

Galvanized by psychoanalysis, psychiatry had completed its long march from rural asylums to Main Street and had completed its evolution from alienists to analysts to activists. Yet despite all the hype, little was or could be done to alleviate the symptoms and suffering of people living with the day-to-day chaos of severe mental illness. Schizophrenics weren't getting better. Manic-depressives weren't getting better. Anxious, autistic, obsessive, and suicidal individuals weren't getting better. For all of its prodigious claims, psychiatry's results fell far short of its promises. What good was psychiatry if it couldn't help those who were most in need?

The rest of medicine was fully aware of psychiatry's impotence and its closed-off, self-referential universe. Physicians from other disciplines looked upon psychiatrists with attitudes ranging from bemusement to open derision. Psychiatry was widely perceived as a haven for ne'er-do-wells, hucksters, and troubled students with their own mental issues, a perception not limited to medical professionals. Vladimir Nabokov summed up the attitude of many skeptics when he wrote, "Let the credulous and the vulgar continue to believe that all mental woes can be cured by a daily application of old Greek myths to their private parts."

As psychoanalysis approached its zenith in the late 1950s, psychiatry was careening off course, as oblivious to danger as an intoxicated driver asleep at the wheel. In retrospect, it is easy to see why American psychiatry veered so wildly astray: It was guided by a mangled map of mental illness.

Chapter 3

What Is Mental Illness?: A Farrago of Diagnoses

The statistics on sanity are that one out of every four Americans is suffering from some form of mental illness. Think of your three best friends. If they're okay, then it's you.

— RITA MAE BROWN

To define illness and health is an almost impossible task. We can define mental illness as being a certain state of existence which is uncomfortable to someone. The suffering may be in the afflicted person or those around him or both.

— PSYCHOANALYST KARL MENNINGER, *THE VITAL BALANCE: THE LIFE PROCESS IN MENTAL HEALTH AND ILLNESS*

The Most Important Three Letters in Psychiatry

If you have ever visited a mental health professional you have probably come across the letters D, S, and M, an acronym for the archaically titled *Diagnostic and Statistical Manual of Mental Disorders.* This authoritative compendium of all known mental illnesses is known as the Bible of Psychiatry, and for good reason—each and every hallowed diagnosis of psychiatry is inscribed within its pages. What you may not realize is that the *DSM* might just be the most influential book written in the past century.

Its contents directly affect how tens of millions of people work, learn, and live—and whether they go to jail. It serves as a career manual for millions of mental health profession-als including psychiatrists, psychologists, social workers, and psychiatric nurses. It dictates the payment of hundreds of billions of dollars to hospitals, physicians, pharmacies, and laboratories by Medicare, Medicaid, and private insurance companies. Applications for academic research funding are granted or denied depending on their use of the manual's diagnostic criteria, and it stimulates (or stifles) tens of billions of dollars' worth of pharmaceutical research and development. Thousands of programs in hospitals, clinics, offices, schools, colleges, prisons, nursing homes, and community centers depend upon its classifications. The *DSM* mandates the accommodations that must be made by employers for mentally disabled workers, and defines workers' compensation claims for mental illnesses. Lawyers, judges, and prison officials use the manual to determine criminal responsibility and tort damages in legal proceedings. Parents can obtain free educational services for their child or special classroom privileges if they claim one of its pediatric diagnoses.

But the *Manual*'s greatest impact is on the lives of tens of millions of men and women who long for relief from the anguish of mental disorder, since first and foremost, the book precisely defines every known mental illness. It is these detailed definitions that empower the *DSM*'s unparalleled medical influence over society.

So how did we get here? How did we go from the psychoanalytical definitions of schizophrenogenic mothers and unconscious neuroses to *DSM* diagnoses ranging from Schizoaffective Disorder, Depressive Type (code 295.70) to Trichotillomania, hair-pulling disorder (code 312.39)? And how can we be confident that our twenty-first-century definitions of mental illness are any better than those inspired by Freud? As we shall see, the stories of psychoanalysis and the *DSM* ran parallel for almost a century before colliding in a tectonic battle for the very soul of psychiatry, a battle waged over the definition of mental illness.

We can trace the primordial origins of the Bible of Psychiatry back to 1840, the first year that the American Census Bureau collected official data on mental illness. The United States was barely fifty years old. Mesmer was not long dead, Freud was not yet born, and virtually every American psychiatrist was an alienist. The United States was obsessed with the statistical enumeration of its citizens through a Constitution-mandated once-a-decade census. The 1830 Census counted disabilities for the first time, though limiting the definition of disability to deafness and blindness. The 1840 Census added a new disability—mental illness—which was tabulated by means of a single checkbox labeled "insane and idiotic."

All the myriad mental and developmental disorders were lumped together within this broad category, and no instructions were provided to the U.S. Marshals tasked with collecting census data for determining whether a citizen should have her "insane and idiotic" box checked off. Based on the prevailing ideas at the time, the census makers probably considered "insanity" to be any mental disturbance severe enough to warrant institutionalization, encompassing what we would now consider schizophrenia, bipolar disorder, depression, and dementia. Similarly, "idiocy" likely referred to any reduced level of intellectual function, which today we would subdivide into Down syndrome, autism, Fragile X syndrome, cretinism, and other conditions. But without any clear guidance, each marshal ended up with his own idiosyncratic notion of what constituted a mental disability—notions that were often influenced by outright racism.

"The most glaring and remarkable errors are found in the Census statements respecting the prevalence of insanity, blindness, deafness, and dumbness, among the people of this nation," the American Statistical Association informed the House of Representatives in 1843, in perhaps the earliest example of a civil protest against excessive labeling of mental illness. "In many towns, all the colored population are stated to be insane; in very many others, two-thirds, one-third, one-fourth or one-tenth of this ill-starred race are reported to be thus afflicted. Moreover, the errors of the census are just as certain in regard to insanity among the whites." Even more troubling was the fact that the results of this census were used to defend slavery: Since the reported rates of insanity and idiocy among African Americans in the Northern states were much higher than in the Southern states, advocates of slavery argued that slavery had mental health benefits.

Amazingly, the same elementary separation of mental conditions into insanity and idiocy remains to this day in our modern institutions. As I write this, every state has a separate administrative infrastructure for mental illness and for developmental disability, despite the fact that each of these conditions affects similar brain structures and mental functions. This somewhat arbitrary division reflects historic and cultural influences on our perception of these conditions rather than any scientifically justified reality. A similarly artificial categorization has resulted in services for substance-use disorders often being administered by a separate government agency and infrastructure, even though addiction disorders are treated by medical science no differently than any other illness.

By the twentieth century, the census had begun to focus attention on gathering statistics on inmates in mental institutions, since it was believed that most of the mentally ill could be found there. But every institution had its own system for categorizing patients, so statistics on mental illness remained highly inconsistent and deeply subjective. In response to this cacophony of classification systems, in 1917 the American Medico-Psychological Association (the forerunner of the American Psychiatric Association) charged its Committee on Statistics with establishing a uniform system for collecting and reporting data from all the mental institutions of America.

The committee, which was comprised of practicing alienists rather than researchers or theorists, relied on their clinical consensus to categorize mental illness into twenty-two "groups," such as "psychosis with brain tumor," "psychosis from syphilis," and "psychosis from senility." The resulting system was published as a slender volume titled *The Statistical Manual for the Use of Institutions for the Insane,* though psychiatrists quickly took to calling it the *Standard.*

For the next three decades, the *Standard* became the most widely used compendium of mental illnesses in the United States, though its sole purpose was to gather statistics on patients in asylums; the *Standard* was not intended (or used) for the diagnosis of outpatients in psychiatrists' offices. The *Standard* was the direct forerunner to the *Diagnostic and Statistical Manual of Mental Illness,* which would eventually lift the phrase "Statistical Manual" from the *Standard,* a phrase that had in turn been borrowed from the language of nineteenth-century census-taking.

Despite the existence of the *Standard,* in the early twentieth century there was nothing approaching consensus on the basic categories of mental illness. Each large psychiatric teaching center employed its own diagnostic system that fulfilled its local needs; psychoses were defined differently in New York than in Chicago or San Francisco. This resulted in a polyglot of names, symptoms, and purported causes for disorders that thwarted professional communication, scholarly research, and the collection of accurate medical data.

Things took a different course on the other side of the Atlantic. Until the latter part of the nineteenth century, there was disarray in European classification of mental illness just as there was in American psychiatry. Then, out of this chaos arose a classifier *par excellence*, a German psychiatrist who imposed rigorous order upon psychiatric diagnosis on the Continent. His influence over the world's conception and diagnosis of mental illness would eventually rival—and then surpass—that of Sigmund Freud.

He Decorates Himself in a Wonderful Way

Emil Kraepelin was born in Germany in 1856—the same year as Freud, and just a few hundred miles from Freud's birthplace. (So many pivotal figures in psychiatry came from German-speaking countries—Franz Mesmer, Wilhelm Griesinger, Sigmund Freud, Emil Kraepelin, Julius Wagner-Jauregg, Manfred Sakel, Eric Kandel—that psychiatry could justifiably be called "the German discipline.") Kraepelin trained in medical school under Paul Fleischig, a famed neuropathologist, and Wilhelm Wundt, the founder of experimental psychology. Under the tutelage of these two empiricists, Kraepelin developed a lifelong appreciation for the value of research and hard evidence.

After becoming a professor of psychiatry in modern-day Estonia, Kraepelin became appalled by the spider's nest of diagnostic terminology and struggled to find some sensible way to bring consistency and order to the classification of mental illness. One of the most vexing problems was the fact that many disorders that seemed distinct often shared some of the same symptoms. For example, anxiety manifested as a prominent symptom of depression and hysteria, while delusions were present in psychosis, mania, and severe forms of depression. Such overlap led many psychiatrists to braid depression and hysteria together as a single disorder, or endorse a single definition that encompassed both psychosis and mania.

Kraepelin was confident that observable symptoms were essential to discriminating mental illnesses, but he didn't think symptoms were enough. (To do so would be akin to grouping all illnesses associated with fever under a single diagnosis.) Consequently, he sought some other criteria that could help distinguish disorders, and by tracking the progress of his patients for their entire lives he found one. Kraepelin decided to organize illnesses not just by symptoms alone but also according to the course of each illness. For example, some psychoses waxed and waned and eventually lifted for no discernible reason, while other psychoses grew worse and worse until afflicted patients became incapable of caring for themselves. In 1883, Kraepelin assembled a draft of his ad hoc classification system in a small book entitled *Compendium der Psychiatrie*.

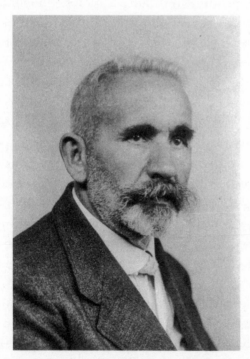

Emil Kraepelin, the founder of the modern system of psychiatric diagnosis. (©National Library of Medicine/Science Source)

In his compendium, Kraepelin divided the psychoses into three groups based upon their life histories: dementia praecox, manic-depressive insanity, and paranoia. Dementia praecox most closely resembled what we would today call schizophrenia, though Kraepelin limited this diagnosis to patients whose intellectual capacity steadily deteriorated over time. Manic-depressive insanity maps onto the modern conception of bipolar disorder. Kraepelin's classification scheme was immediately marked by controversy because dementia praecox and manic-depressive illness had usually been considered manifestations of the same underlying disorder, though Kraepelin justified the distinction by pointing out that manic-depressive illness was episodic rather than continuous, like dementia praecox.

Despite the initial resistance to Kraepelin's novel proposal, his classification system was eventually accepted by the majority of European psychiatrists, and by the 1890s it had become the first common language used by European psychiatrists of all theoretical bents to discuss the psychoses. To help explain his classification system, Kraepelin wrote portraits of prototypical cases for each diagnosis, derived from his own experiences with patients. These vivid portraits became a pedagogical device that influenced generations of European psychiatrists and are as compelling today as when he wrote them more than a century ago. His detailed accounts of dementia praecox and manic-depressive illness even persuaded many psychiatrists that the two conditions were distinct. Here is an excerpt from his description of dementia praecox:

> The patients see mice, ants, the hound of hell, scythes, and axes. They hear cocks crowing, shooting, birds chirping, spirits knockings, bees humming, murmurings, screaming, scolding, voices from the cellar. The voices say: "That man

must be beheaded, hanged," "Swine, wicked wretch, you will be done for." The patient is the greatest sinner, has denied God, God has forsaken him, he is eternally lost, he is going to hell. The patient notices that he is looked at in a peculiar way, laughed at, scoffed at, that people are jeering at him. People spy on him; Jews, anarchists, spiritualists, persecute him; they poison the atmosphere with toxic powder, the beer with prussic acid.

And of manic-depressive psychosis:

The patient is a stranger to fatigue, his activity goes on day and night; ideas flow to him. The patient changes his furniture, visits distant acquaintances. Politics, the universal language, aeronautics, the women's question, public affairs of all kinds and their need for improvement, gives him employment. He has 16,000 picture post-cards of his little village printed. He cannot be silent for long. The patient boasts about his prospects of marriage, gives himself out as a count, speaks of inheritances which he may expect, has visiting cards printed with a crown on them. He can take the place of many a professor or diplomatist. The patient sings, chatters, dances, romps about, does gymnastics, beats time, claps his hands, scolds, threatens, throws everything down on the floor, undresses, decorates himself in a wonderful way.

Over the following decade, Kraepelin's hastily written compendium swelled into a wildly popular textbook. New editions came out with increasing frequency, each larger than the last. By the 1930s, a majority of European psychiatrists had embraced Kraepelin's classifications. Across the Atlantic, by contrast, it was a very different story. While a minority of

American alienists had adopted his system of diagnosis in the early decades of the twentieth century, by the end of World War II his influence on American psychiatry had been almost completely wiped out by the rise of the Freudians, at precisely the same time that Freudian influence in Europe was being expunged by the Nazis.

Infinite Neuroses

According to psychoanalytical doctrine, since mental illness emanated from a person's unique unconscious conflicts, it was infinitely variable and could not be neatly packed into diagnostic boxes. Each case must be treated (and diagnosed) on its own merits. Kraepelin, on the contrary, drew a sharp boundary between mental health and mental illness. This bright dividing line, along with his system of classifying disorders based on their symptoms and time-course of the illness, ran entirely counter to the psychoanalytic conception of mental disease, which held that a person's mental state lay on a continuum between psychopathology and sanity; everyone possessed some degree of mental dysfunction, said the Freudians.

Freud himself acknowledged general patterns of dysfunctional behavior—like hysteria, obsessiveness, phobias, anxiety, depression—but he believed they were all mutable manifestations of neuroses that grew out of emotional stresses occurring at specific stages of development. For example, a psychoanalytic diagnosis of Abigail Abercrombie might account for her spells of anxiety by connecting them to the way she reacted to her parents' strict Lutheran upbringing, combined with her decision to leave home at an early age to work rather than marry. A Kraepelinian diagnosis would characterize Abbey as suffering from an anxiety disorder based upon her symptoms of intense fear and discomfort accompanied by heart palpitations, sweating, and dizziness, symptoms that occurred together in regular episodes. (Wilhelm Reich's diagnostic method presents yet another contrast: He claimed that the physical constriction of Abbey's body impeded the free flow of her orgones, which caused her anxiety.) These are strikingly different interpretations.

Psychoanalysts believed that attending too much to a patient's specific symptoms could be a distraction, leading the psychiatrist away from the true nature of a disorder. The proper role for the psychoanalyst was to look beyond mere behaviors, symptomatic or otherwise, to unearth the hidden emotional dynamics and historical narrative of a patient's life. Given this profound discordance in the basic conceptualization of mental illness within Freud's and Kraepelin's systems, you may not be surprised to learn that Emil Kraepelin was openly derisive of psychoanalysis:

> We meet everywhere the characteristic features of Freudian investigation, the representation of arbitrary assumptions and conjectures as assured facts, which are used without hesitation for the building up of new castles in the air towering ever higher, and the tendency to generalization beyond all measure from a single observation. As I am more accustomed to walking upon the surer foundations of direct experience, my Philistine conscience of natural science stumbles at every step upon objections, uncertainties, and doubts, while Freud's disciples' soaring tower of imagination carries them over without difficulty.

To complicate matters further, practitioners in each individual school of psychoanalysis had their own categories and definitions of unconscious conflicts. Strict Freudians emphasized the central role of sexual conflicts. Adlerians identified aggression as the key source of conflict. The school of ego psychology combined these approaches, focusing on both sexual and aggressive drives. Jungians, meanwhile, sought to identify the clash of psychic archetypes within a person's unconscious.

Other psychoanalysts simply invented their own diagnoses out of whole cloth. Helene Deutsch, a renowned Austrian émigré, created the "as if personality" to describe people "who seem normal enough because they substituted pseudo-emotional contacts for real connections to other people; they behave 'as if' they had feelings and relations with other people rather than superficial pseudo-relations." Paul Hoch and Phillip Polatin proposed "pseudoneurotic schizophrenia" to describe people who invested their relationships with too little — or perhaps too much — emotional attachment. It is chilling to think that patients diagnosed with pseudoneurotic schizophrenia were once referred to the psychosurgery clinic here at Columbia University, where Hoch worked.

Freud contributed his fair share of psychopathological creations, such as the anal-retentive personality disorder: "an anal-erotic character style characterized by orderliness, parsimony, and obstinacy." Someone who excessively consumed food, alcohol, or drugs was labeled an oral-dependent personality by Freud, who argued that such patients had been deprived of oral nourishment as infants (namely, breast-feeding). Freud characterized other neurotic conflicts as Oedipal complexes (a man unconsciously wanting to kill his father and have sex with his mother), Electra complexes (a woman unconsciously wanting to kill her mother and have sex with her father), castration anxiety (a boy fearing losing his penis as punishment for his sexual attraction to his mother), or penis envy (a woman unconsciously longing for the power and status afforded by a penis).

The most notorious psychoanalytic diagnosis was undoubtedly homosexuality. In an era when society considered homosexuality both immoral and illegal, psychiatry labeled it a mental disorder as well. Ironically, Freud himself did not believe that homosexuality was a mental illness, and was supportive of homosexual acquaintances in letters and personal interactions. But from the 1940s to the 1970s, the leading psychoanalytical view of homosexuality held that it developed in the first two years of life due to a controlling mother who prevented her son from separating from her, and a weak or rejecting father who did not serve as a role model for his son or support his efforts to escape from the mother.

This unfounded and immensely destructive attribution of unconscious conflicts in homosexual persons illustrates the broad fallibility and potential for misuse of the psychoanalytic approach to diagnosis. In the absence of a rigorous scientific methodology, therapists were prone to projecting their own values and intuitions onto the mental lives of their patients. At the start of World War II, each psychoanalyst clung to his own ideas about what constituted a psychic conflict and how to identify one. As Kraepelin's ideas were bringing order to the European classification of mental illness, American diagnosis remained a raucous farrago of diagnoses.

It was the American military that finally came to psychiatry's aid.

Psychotic Soldiers

As the American military recruited ever-increasing numbers of soldiers to fight in the Second World War, it encountered a puzzling problem. Each potential recruit was evaluated by a military doctor to determine if he was fit to serve. Military officials expected that the rates of rejection for medical reasons would be consistent from state to state, but when they reviewed the actual rejection rates around the country, they were surprised to find that the rejection rates varied wildly. A draft board in Wichita might have a 20 percent rejection rate, while a draft board in Baltimore might reject 60 percent of its applicants. When military officials looked more closely at the problem, they realized that this variability was not due to physical conditions, such as flat feet or heart murmurs, it was due to dramatic differences in the way each doctor judged recruits to be mentally ill.

The military had not considered the consequences of applying contemporary methods of psychiatric diagnosis to the evaluation of conscripted soldiers. If a military doctor found a potential recruit unfit for service, he needed to specify the precise diagnosis that rendered the draftee ineligible... but, of course, Freud-influenced psychiatrists were not used to establishing precise diagnoses. Each psychoanalytical psychiatrist employed his own idiosyncratic interpretation of buried conflicts and neuroses. Even non-Freudians could not refer to an obvious diagnostic system to use to justify their rejections. While many non-Freudians relied on the *Standard*, that manual had been developed to gather statistics on institutionalized patients; it was never designed to diagnose mental illnesses that might be found in the wider community, and it was certainly never intended to evaluate the ability of potential soldiers to function in combat.

Recruits who exhibited behavior that was perceived as problematic in a military setting—such as an inability to pay attention or hostility toward authority—were often shoehorned into a category like "Psychopathic Personality." Some draft boards saw as many as 40 percent of volunteers rejected because of "psychosis."

In hopes of establishing a consistent and comprehensive system for evaluating the mental health of potential recruits, the army convened a committee in 1941 headed by William

Menninger, former president of the American Psychiatric Association and cofounder of the Menninger Clinic, to develop a set of clearly defined diagnoses for mental illness that could be used to determine whether a given candidate was fit to serve. (Ironically, William's brother Karl, who cofounded the Menninger Clinic, wrote in his book *The Vital Balance,* "There is only one class of mental illness—namely, mental illness. Thus, diagnostic nomenclature is not only useless but restrictive and obstructive.")

Menninger issued his new psychiatric classification system in 1943 as a twenty-eight-page War Department Technical Bulletin that became known as the *Medical 203,* after its bulletin number. It was immediately implemented as the official manual for diagnosing both recruits and soldiers in the American military. The *Medical 203* described about sixty disorders and represented a landmark in clinical psychiatry: It was the first diagnostic system that classified every known form of mental illness, including serious disorders found in patients in mental institutions and mild neuroses found in patients who could function effectively in society.

At last, here was a comprehensive roadmap for diagnosing mental illness—and yet the *Medical 203* was almost completely ignored by civilian psychiatrists. For shrinks seeing patients in their private practices, the prevailing sentiment was, "I didn't need a pointless classification manual before the war, and I certainly don't need one now." Psychoanalysts continued to use their own creative diagnoses, while asylum psychiatrists and teaching centers continued to rely on the *Standard* or some local variant.

After the war ended, American psychiatry remained a patchwork of diagnostic systems. Imagine a medical world where military physicians defined heart attacks one way, universities defined heart attacks another way, hospitals defined them yet another way, while primary care physicians suggested that since everybody's heart was sick to some degree, heart attacks didn't really exist at all. American psychiatry was experiencing a crisis of reliability.

In a famous study in 1949, three psychiatrists independently interviewed the same thirty-five patients and independently came up with their own diagnosis for each patient. They ended up agreeing on the same diagnosis for a given patient (such as "manic-depressive illness") only 20 percent of the time. (Consider how frustrated you might feel if oncologists only agreed that the mole on your arm was skin cancer 20 percent of the time.) The leaders of the American Psychiatric Association recognized that this unsettling lack of reliability would eventually undermine the public credibility of psychiatry. Despite the protestations of many psychoanalysts, in 1950 the APA formed a Committee on Nomenclature and Statistics tasked with the development of a diagnostic system that would standardize the classification of mental illness within civilian psychiatry once and for all. Unlike the *Standard*, this new system would include diagnoses relevant to private practice, the illnesses that shrinks saw (or believed they saw) every day in their offices.

The committee took the *Medical 203* as its starting point, lifting many passages of text directly from Menninger's military bulletin. At the same time, the committee also sought to establish continuity with the *Standard* by borrowing the phrase "Statistical Manual" from its title. In 1952, the APA published the new system as the very first *Diagnostic and Statistical Manual of Mental Disorders*, today known as the *DSM-I*. It listed 106 mental disorders—an expansion from the 22 disorders in the *Standard* and the 60 disorders in the *Medical 203*. It relied heavily on psychoanalytical concepts, most obviously in the names of disorders, which were referred to as "reactions," a term originating with the psychoanalyst Adolf Meyer, who oversaw the creation of the *DSM-I* while he was president of the APA and who believed that mental illness arose from maladaptive habits in response to the stressors of life. According to Meyer, mental illness should be diagnosed by identifying a patient's unique stressors and the patient's responses to them. Schizophrenia, for example, was a bundle of unruly reactions to the stresses and challenges of life. This perspective was codified in the *DSM-I*'s description of psychotic reactions: "a psychotic reaction may be defined as one in which the personality, in its struggle for adjustment to internal and external stresses, utilizes severe affective disturbance, profound autism and withdrawal from reality, and/or formation of delusions or hallucinations."

For a medical specialty that had splintered into an anarchy of institution-specific definitions of illness, at last there was a single unifying document that could be used in any psychiatric setting, whether in an Arkansas state mental institution, an analyst's office on the Upper East Side of Manhattan, or a medical unit on the front lines in Korea. The *DSM-I* represented a necessary first step in the unification and standardization of psychiatric medicine.

But it was also a precarious first step, since none of the diagnoses in the *DSM-I* were based upon scientific evidence or empirical research. They reflected the consensus of a committee that mostly consisted of practicing psychoanalysts, rather than researchers. It would not be long before the egregious shortcomings of the *DSM* would be exposed for the entire world to see.

On Being Sane in Insane Places

By the time I started medical school in 1970, the second edition of the *DSM* was in use. *DSM-II* was a rather thin spiral-bound paperback that cost $3.50. It had been published in 1968 to little fanfare, contained 182 disorders (almost double the number in *DSM-I*), and was every bit as vague and inconsistent as its predecessor. *DSM-II* had dropped the term *reactions* but retained the term *neuroses*. I only learned these facts later; while I was in medical school, I hardly laid eyes on the *DSM-II*— and neither did most psychiatry and psychology trainees.

Instead, I invested in an expensive black tome titled *The Comprehensive Textbook of Psychiatry*, a far more common reference book. This volume contained a potpourri of information from anthropology, sociology, and psychology—all mixed together with a heavy dose of psychoanalytic theory, of course. It still contained chapters on sleep therapy, insulin coma therapy, and lobotomies, while only 130 of its 1,600 pages contained references to the brain or neuroscience.

Most of what we learned in medical school did not come from books but from our instructors, each of whom purveyed his own interpretation of psychiatric diagnosis. One day, after we interviewed a young man who was manifestly psychotic, my professor began discussing the patient's characteristics by way of formulating his diagnosis. In doing so he declared that the patient had the characteristic "smell of schizophrenia." At first I thought he was using scent as a metaphor, like you might refer to the "sweet smell of success." Eventually I realized that, like a psychiatric bloodhound, he believed his refined nose and olfaction could detect the apparently rather earthy aroma of the schizophrenic.

Other professors improvised their own methods of diagnosis like jazz musicians riffing on a melody, and encouraged us to follow their lead. Although this approach certainly respected the individual concerns and experiences of each patient—and liberated a clinician's creativity—it did not foster diagnostic consistency. Confusing an impressionable young psychiatrist still further was a bevy of diagnostic frameworks that had splintered from Freudian theory: Adlerian, Jungian, Sullivanian, Kleinian, Kohutian, and many others, each coming from creative thinkers who were persuasive orators and charismatic personalities. It was as if the professional influence of each new diagnostic model radiated directly out of the dash and verve of its creator's persona, rather than arising from any scientific discovery or body of evidence. When it came to clinical sway in the 1970s, the *DSM* was completely eclipsed by its cultish competitors.

Most shrinks, of course, didn't view this as a problem. So what if there was an anarchy of philosophies about mental illness—that means I'm free to choose the one that best suits my own style! There was very little in the way of accountability and even less concern that the profession lacked anything that remotely resembled a set of "best practices." This complacent attitude would be shattered by a study that slammed into psychiatry with the force of a battering ram.

In 1973 a sensational exposé appeared in the normally staid columns of the prestigious journal *Science.* A few pages after papers with technical titles like "Earliest Radiocarbon Dates for Domesticated Animals" and "Gene Flow and Population Differentiation" came a real attention-grabber: "On Being Sane in Insane Places." The author was David Rosenhan. He was a little-known Stanford-trained lawyer who had recently obtained a psychology degree but lacked any clinical experience. His very first sentence made it clear that he intended to tackle one of the most basic questions for any medicine that laid claim to the mind: "If sanity and insanity exist, how shall we know them?"

Rosenhan proposed an experiment to determine how American psychiatry answered this question. Suppose perfectly normal people with no history of mental illness were admitted to a mental hospital. Would they be discovered to be sane? If so, how? Rosenhan did not merely offer this up as a thought experiment—he proceeded to share the results of an extraordinary study he had conducted over the previous year.

Unbeknownst to the hospital staffs, Rosenhan had engineered the secret admission of eight sane people to twelve different mental hospitals in five separate states on the East and West Coasts (some of his confederates were admitted to multiple hospitals). These "pseudopatients" used fake identities that varied their age and profession. At each hospital, they telephoned ahead for an appointment, and when they arrived they complained of hearing voices that uttered three words: "empty," "hollow," and "thud."

In every instance, the pseudopatient was voluntarily admitted to the hospital. Once the confederates reached the psychiatry ward, they were instructed to say to the staff that they were no longer hearing voices (though they never shared that they had faked their symptoms to get admitted). They proceeded to act normally, presumably not evincing any symptoms of illness. Their behavior on the wards was variously recorded by nurses as "friendly," "cooperative," and "exhibiting no abnormal indications."

The pretense of Rosenhan's pseudopatients was never detected. All but one was diagnosed as schizophrenic (the outlier was diagnosed as manic-depressive), and when they were discharged all but the manic-depressive patient were labeled as having "schizophrenia in remission." The length of their hospitalizations varied from seven to fifty-two days. Yet, as Rosenhan observed with scorn, no one on the staff ever raised the issue of their apparent sanity. (This assertion is open to debate, since many nurses did record that the pseudopatients were behaving normally.) Rosenhan concluded, "We cannot distinguish the sane from the insane in psychiatric hospitals," and he condemned the entire profession for unreliable diagnoses and excessive labeling. The latter accusation was somewhat ironic, considering that the majority of psychiatrists at the time rejected diagnostic labels in favor of nuanced and individualistic psychoanalytic interpretations.

Rosenhan's *Science* article provoked widespread outrage and derision among both the general public and the medical community, a reaction that took psychiatrists completely by surprise. Their response was defensive. They criticized Rosenhan's study head on, arguing (quite reasonably, in my opinion) that if someone shows up at a mental hospital and complains of hearing voices, the sensible and ethical course of action is to admit her for observation and treatment. After all, schizophrenia can be a dangerous illness. If the psychiatrists did not accept at face value what their patients told them, then not just psychiatry but the entire medical profession would be at risk. If a patient showed up in the emergency room and claimed to have chest pain, but the staff refused to admit her for testing without further proof of her pain, she might die. Similarly, if a person fabricated illness by intentionally swallowing a vial of blood in order to deceive doctors, then induced himself to cough up blood in the emergency room, it would be extremely cynical to declare the doctors incompetent if they performed an endoscopy to find the source of the bleeding.

Rosenhan openly admitted his antipathy toward the psychiatric profession, and on the heels of the outrage provoked by his first study, he saw another opportunity to inflict damage on psychiatry's crumbling credibility. He approached a large prestigious teaching hospital that had been especially vocal in contesting Rosenhan's findings with a new challenge: "Over the coming year, I will send in another round of imposters to your hospital. You try to detect them, knowing full well that they will be coming, and at the end of the year we see how many you catch." The unidentified hospital took the bait, and—perhaps unwisely—agreed to the contest.

Out of 193 new patients evaluated over the course of the ensuing year, the staff identified 41 as potential impersonators. A gleeful Rosenhan then revealed that no imposters had been sent to the hospital. He then declared that, given psychiatry's inability to distinguish the sane from the insane, the profession was doing the medical equivalent of convicting innocent people of crimes and sentencing them to prison.

While most psychiatrists dismissed Rosenhan's study as a self-aggrandizing gimmick, the profession could not escape the embarrassment or ignore the public outcry. Newspapers were filled with op-eds and letters to the editor denouncing psychiatry as a sham and a racket. Even more distressing to psychiatrists, medical colleagues and insurance companies had begun to vocally express their own disillusionment with psychiatry. Following the publication of the Rosenhan study, insurance companies like Aetna and Blue Cross dramatically slashed the mental health benefits in their policies as they became increasingly cognizant of the fact that psychiatric diagnosis and treatment were freewheeling affairs that took place without oversight or accountability. In 1975, the vice president of Blue Cross told *Psychiatric News*, "In psychiatry, compared to other types of medical services, there is less clarity and uniformity of terminology concerning mental diagnoses, treatment modalities, and types of facilities providing care. One dimension of this problem arises from the latent or private nature of many services; only the patient and therapist have direct knowledge of what services were provided and why."

As bad as this was, there was much more to come. The Rosenhan study fueled a rapidly accelerating activist movement that sought to eliminate psychiatry entirely, a movement launched a decade earlier by a man named Thomas Szasz.

The Antipsychiatry Movement and the Great Crisis

In 1961, Thomas Szasz, a Hungarian-born psychiatrist on the faculty of the State University of New York at Syracuse, published a highly influential book that has remained in print to this very day, *The Myth of Mental Illness*. In this book he argues that mental illnesses are not medical realities like diabetes and hypertension, but are fictions invented by psychiatry to justify charging patients for unscientific therapies of unknown effectiveness. Szasz declared that psychiatry was a "pseudo-science" like alchemy and astrology—not an unreasonable critique at a time when psychoanalysis was the cult-like force that dominated psychiatry.

The book won him instant fame, especially among young people who were embracing countercultural values and challenging traditional forms of authority. By the mid-1960s, students flocked to study with him at SUNY. He began publishing articles and giving lectures advocating a new approach to psychotherapy. The true and worthy goal of an analyst, Szasz contended, was to "unravel the game of life that the patient plays." Psychiatrists, therefore, should not assume that there is something "wrong" with odd behavior, a message that resonated with a generation adopting other anti-authoritarian slogans such as "Turn on, Tune in, Drop Out" and "Make Love, Not War."

Szasz's views amounted to a form of behavioral relativism that viewed any unusual behavior as meaningful and valid if viewed from the proper perspective. Szasz might say that Elena Conway's decision to accompany the sleazy middle-aged stranger to his apartment was a valid expression of her plucky personality and her admirable willingness to not judge someone by his appearance, rather than impaired judgment caused by an arbitrary "illness" that doctors called "schizophrenia."

Szasz wanted to completely do away with mental hospitals: "Involuntary mental hospitalization is like slavery. Refining the standards for commitment is like prettifying the slave plantations. The problem is not how to improve commitment, but how to abolish it."

Szasz's ideas helped give birth to an organized activist movement that questioned the very existence of the profession of psychiatry and called for its eradication, and *The Myth of Mental Illness* became its manifesto. Szasz's final betrayal of his profession came in 1969 when he joined L. Ron Hubbard and the Church of Scientology to found the Citizens Commission on Human Rights (CCHR). Explicitly drawing upon Szasz's arguments, the CCHR holds that "so-called mental illness" is not a medical disease, that psychiatric medication is fraudulent and dangerous, and that the psychiatric profession should be condemned.

Szasz served as inspiration for others who doubted the value of psychiatry, including an unknown sociologist named Erving Goffman. In 1961, Goffman published the book *Asylums,* decrying the deplorable conditions in American mental institutions. Since the population of asylums was near its all-time high, there was little question that most of these institutions were oppressive, overcrowded, and bleak. What was Goffman's response to this indisputable social problem? He declared that mental illness did not exist.

According to Goffman, what psychiatrists called mental illness was actually society's failure to understand the motivations of unconventional people; Western society had imposed what he called a "medical mandate over these offenders. Inmates were called patients." Goffman wrote that his goal in investigating mental institutions was "to learn about the social world of the hospital inmate." He intentionally avoided social contact with the staff, declaring that "to describe the patient's situation faithfully is necessarily to present a partisan view." He defended this overt bias by claiming "the imbalance is at least on the right side of the scale, since almost all professional literature on mental patients is written from the point of view of the psychiatrists, and I, socially speaking, am on the other side."

The urge to propound theories of human behavior is a basic human impulse we all frequently indulge in; this may be why so many psychiatric researchers feel compelled to throw aside the theories and research of previous scientists in order to articulate their own Grand Explanation of mental illness. Despite the fact that Goffman was trained in sociology (not psychiatry) and had no clinical experience whatsoever, the urge for propounding his own Grand Explanation of mental illness soon overtook him.

Individuals diagnosed with mental illness did not actually have a legitimate medical condition, insisted Goffman, but were instead the victims of society's reaction to them—what Goffman termed "social influences," such as poverty, society's rejection of their behavior as inappropriate, and proximity to a mental institution. But what if a person was *convinced* that something was wrong with her, as in the case of Abigail Abercrombie and her panic attacks? Goffman replied that her perceptions of her racing heart, her sense of imminent doom, and her feeling of losing control were all shaped by cultural stereotypes of how a person *should* behave when she is anxious.

As Szasz and Goffman were rising in prominence, another antipsychiatry figure emerged on the other side of the Atlantic: the Scottish psychiatrist R. D. Laing. While Laing believed that mental illness existed, like Goffman he placed the source of illness in a person's social environment, especially disruptions in the family network. In particular, Laing considered psychotic behavior an expression of distress prompted by a person's intolerable social circumstances; schizophrenia, to his thinking, was a cry for help.

Laing believed that a therapist could interpret the personal symbolism of a patient's psychosis (shades of Freud's dream interpretations) and use this divination to address the environmental issues that were the true source of the patient's schizophrenia. To successfully decode a patient's psychotic symptomatology, Laing suggested that the therapist should draw upon his own "psychotic possibilities." Only in that way could he comprehend the schizophrenic's "existential position"—"his distinctiveness, and differentness, his separateness and loneliness and despair."

The ideas of Szasz, Laing, and Goffman formed the intellectual underpinnings of a burgeoning antipsychiatry movement that soon joined forces with social activists such as the Black Panthers, Marxists, Vietnam War protesters, and other organizations that encouraged the defiance of the conventions and authority of an oppressive Western society. In 1968, the antipsychiatrists staged their first demonstrations at an annual meeting of the American Psychiatric Association. The following year, at the APA meeting in Miami, delegates looked out the window to discover an airplane circling overhead pulling a banner that read "Psychiatry Kills." Every year since then, APA meetings have been accompanied by the bullhorns and pickets of antipsychiatry protests, including the 2014 meeting in New York, over which I presided.

Despite the kernels of truth in the antipsychiatry movement's arguments in the 1960s and 1970s—such as their quite valid assertion that psychiatric diagnosis was highly unreliable—many of their claims were based on extreme distortions of data or oversimplifications of clinical realities. The most elaborate antipsychiatry critiques tended to emerge from ivory tower intellectuals and political radicals who lacked any direct expe-

THE STORY OF DIAGNOSIS

rience with mental illness, or from clinical mavericks who operated on the fringes of clinical psychiatry...and who may not have even believed the ideas they were touting.

Dr. Fuller Torrey, a prominent schizophrenia researcher and leading public spokesperson for mental illness, told me, "Laing's convictions were eventually put to the test when his own daughter developed schizophrenia. After that, he became disillusioned with his own ideas. People who knew Laing told me that he became a guy asking for money by giving lectures on ideas he no longer believed in. Same with Szasz, who I met several times. He made it pretty clear he understood that schizophrenia qualified as a true brain disease, but he was never going to say so publicly."

The antipsychiatry movement continues to harm the very individuals it purports to be helping—namely, the mentally ill. Aside from Laing, the leading figures of antipsychiatry blithely ignored the issue of human suffering, suggesting that a depressed person's misery or a paranoid schizophrenic's feelings of persecution would dissipate if we merely respected and supported their atypical beliefs. They also ignored the danger that schizophrenics sometimes presented to others.

The eminent psychiatrist Aaron Beck shared with me one example of the true cost of such ignorance. "I had been treating a potentially homicidal inpatient who made contact with Thomas Szasz, who then put direct pressure on the Pennsylvania Hospital to discharge the patient. After he was released, the patient was responsible for several murders and was only stopped when his wife, whom he threatened to kill, shot him. I think that the 'myth of mental illness' promulgated by Szasz was not only absurd but also damaging to the patients themselves."

State governments, which were always eyeing ways to cut funding for the mentally ill (especially state mental institutions, usually one of the most expensive line items in any state budget), were only too happy to give credence to antipsychiatry arguments. While purporting to adopt humane postures, they cited Szasz, Laing, and Goffman as scientific and moral justification for emptying out the state asylums and dumping patients back into the community. While legislators were able to save money in their budgets, many patients in these asylums were elderly and in poor health and had nowhere else to go. This ill-conceived policy of deinstitutionalization directly contributed to the epidemic of homelessness, many of whom were mentally ill, and the rapid growth of the mentally ill population in prisons, which persists to this day. Insurance companies also readily accepted the antipsychiatrists' argument that mental illness was simply a "problem in living" and not a medical condition and therefore treatment for such "illnesses" should not be reimbursed, leading to even more cutbacks in coverage.

The final and most enduring professional blow that resulted from the antipsychiatry movement was an assault on psychiatry's near-monopoly of therapeutic treatment. Since the core argument of the antipsychiatry movement was that mental illness was not a medical condition but a social problem, psychiatrists could no longer claim they should be the sole medical overseers of mental health care. Clinical psychologists, social workers, pastoral counselors, new age practitioners, encounter groups, and other lay therapists leveraged the antipsychiatrists' arguments to strengthen their own legitimacy as providers for the mentally ill, diverting increasing numbers of patients from medically trained psychiatrists. Soon, proliferating numbers of self-styled therapists without any license at all began carving up the mental health care market. The most ominous and aggressive of these non-medical alternative therapies was the Church of Scientology, a quasi-religious system of beliefs created by the science fiction writer L. Ron Hubbard. Scientology holds that people are immortal beings who have forgotten their true nature and past lives. They condemn the use of psychiatric drugs, instead encouraging individuals to undergo a process of "auditing" whereby they consciously re-experience painful or traumatic events from their past in order to free themselves from their harmful effects.

Each of the rival groups espoused its own theories and methods, but all shared a common conviction articulated so emphatically by the antipsychiatrists: Mental disorders were not bona fide medical illnesses and therefore did not need to be treated by physicians. The Conways, who brought their schizophrenic daughter Elena to see me, are an example of those who embrace the arguments of the antipsychiatrists, favoring holistic treatments over medical ones.

By the mid-1970s, American psychiatry was being battered on every front. Academics, lawyers, activists, artists, and even psychiatrists were publicly condemning the profession on a regular basis. The 1975 movie *One Flew Over the Cuckoo's Nest*, based on Ken Kesey's 1962 hit novel, came to symbolize the surging sentiment against psychiatry. This Academy Award–winning film was set in an Oregon state mental institution where the main character, a charismatic and mischievous rogue played by Jack Nicholson, was hospitalized for antisocial behavior. Nicholson leads a boisterous patient rebellion against the tyrannical authority of the psychiatric ward, Nurse Ratched, who cruelly reasserts control by forcing McMurphy to undergo electroshock treatment and then having him lobotomized. While the story was intended as a political allegory rather than an antipsychiatry polemic, the film emblazoned the image of a morally and scientifically bankrupt profession upon the public's mind.

Surveying the situation in the early 1970s, the American Psychiatric Association warned its members, "Our profession has been brought to the edge of extinction." The Board of Trustees called an emergency conference in February of 1973 to consider how to address the crisis and counter the rampant criticism. Everyone agreed that there was one fundamental problem central to all of psychiatry's troubles: It still had no reliable, *scientific* method for diagnosing mental illness.

Chapter 4

Destroying the Rembrandts, Goyas, and Van Goghs: Anti-Freudians to the Rescue

Physicians think they do a lot for a patient when they give his disease a name.

— IMMANUEL KANT

Unfortunately for us all, the DSM-III *in its present version would seem to have all the earmarks for causing an upheaval in American psychiatry which will not soon be put down.*
— BOYD L. BURRIS, PRESIDENT OF THE BALTIMORE WASHINGTON SOCIETY FOR PSYCHOANALYSIS, 1979

An Unlikely Hero

There was little in the early life of Robert Leopold Spitzer to suggest he would one day be a psychiatric revolutionary, but it wasn't hard to find indications of a methodical approach to human behavior. "When I was twelve years old I went to summer camp for two months, and I developed considerable interest in some of the female campers," Spitzer tells me. "So I made a graph on the wall of my feelings towards five or six girls. I charted my feelings as they went up and down over the course of summer camp. I also recall being bothered by the fact that I was attracted to girls that I didn't really *like* very much, so maybe my graph helped me make sense of my feelings."

At age fifteen, Spitzer asked his parents for permission to try therapy with an acolyte of Wilhelm Reich. He thought that it might help him understand girls better. His parents refused—they believed, rather perceptively, that Reich's orgonomy was a sham. Undeterred, Spitzer snuck out of his apartment and secretly attended sessions, paying five dollars a week to a Reichian therapist in downtown Manhattan. The therapist, a young man, followed Reich's practice of physically manipulating the body and spent the sessions pushing Spitzer's limbs around without talking very much. Spitzer does remember one thing the therapist told him. "If I freed myself of my crippling inhibitions, I would experience a physical streaming, a heightened sense of awareness in my body."

Seeking that sense of "streaming," Spitzer persuaded a Reichian analyst who possessed an orgone accumulator to allow him to use the device. He spent many hours sitting within the booth's narrow wooden walls patiently absorbing the invisible orgone energy that he hoped would make him a happier, stronger, smarter person. But after a year of Reichian therapy and treatments, Spitzer grew disillusioned with orgonomy. And, like many zealots who lose their faith, he became determined to unmask and expose his former orthodoxy.

In 1953, during his final year as a Cornell University undergraduate, Spitzer devised eight experiments to test Reich's claims about the existence of orgone energy. For some trials, he enlisted students to serve as subjects. For other experiments, he served as his own subject. After completing all eight experiments, Spitzer concluded that "careful examination of the data in no way proves or even hints at the existence of orgone energy."

Most undergraduate research never reaches an audience wider than the student's own advisor, and Spitzer's study was no exception; when he submitted his paper debunking orgonomy to the *American Journal of Psychiatry*, the editors promptly rejected it. But a few months later he received an unexpected visitor to his dorm room: an official from the Food and Drug

Administration (FDA). The man explained that the FDA was investigating Reich's claims of curing cancer. They were looking for an expert witness to testify about the effectiveness of Reich's orgone accumulators—or lack thereof—and they had obtained Spitzer's name from the American Psychiatric Association, the publisher of the *American Journal of Psychiatry*. Would Spitzer be interested? It was a gratifying response for an aspiring young scientist, though in the end Spitzer's testimony was not needed. The incident demonstrated that Spitzer was already prepared to challenge psychiatric authority using evidence and reason.

After graduating from the New York University School of Medicine in 1957, Spitzer began his training in psychiatry at Columbia University and psychoanalysis in its Center for Psychoanalytic Training and Research, the most influential psychoanalytic institute in America. But once Spitzer started treating his own patients using psychoanalysis, he soon became disillusioned once again. Despite his ardent efforts to properly apply the nuances and convolutions of psychoanalytical theory, his patients rarely seemed to improve. Spitzer says, "As time went on, I became more aware that I couldn't be confident I was telling them anything more than what I wanted to believe. I was trying to convince them they could change, but I wasn't sure that was true."

Spitzer soldiered on as a young Columbia University clinician, hoping that he would encounter some opportunity to change the course of his career. In 1966, that opportunity arrived in the Columbia University cafeteria. Spitzer shared a lunch table with Ernest Gruenberg, a senior Columbia faculty member and the chair of the Task Force for the *DSM-II*, which was under development. Gruenberg knew Spitzer from around the department and had always liked him, and the two men enjoyed an easy and lively conversation. By the time they finished their sandwiches, Gruenberg made the young man an offer: "We're almost done with the

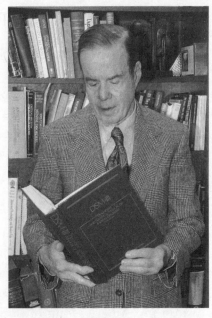

Robert Spitzer, the architect of *DSM-III*. (Courtesy of Eve Vagg, New York State Psychiatric Institute)

DSM-II, but I still need somebody to take notes and do a little editing. Would you be interested?"

Spitzer asked if he would be paid. Gruenberg smiled and shook his head. "Nope," he replied. Spitzer shrugged and said, "I'll take the job."

The *DSM* was still considered useless by the vast majority of psychiatrists, and nobody viewed the bureaucratic cataloging of diagnoses as a stepping-stone toward career advancement. But Spitzer thought he would enjoy the intellectual puzzle of carving apart mental illnesses more than the vague and inconclusive process of psychoanalysis. His enthusiasm and diligence as the *DSM-II* scribe was quickly rewarded by his promotion to an official position as a full-fledged member of the Task Force, making him at age thirty-four the youngest member of the *DSM-II* team.

After the new edition of the *Manual* was completed, Spitzer continued to serve as a member of the APA's soporifically titled Committee on Nomenclature and Statistics. Under most circumstances, this was a humdrum position with little professional upside, and Spitzer had zero expectation that his involvement would lead anywhere—until controversy abruptly thrust him into the national spotlight: the battle over the *DSM* diagnosis of homosexuality.

Classifying Homosexuality

American psychiatry had long considered homosexuality to represent deviant behavior, and generations of psychiatrists had labeled it a mental disorder. *DSM-I* described homosexuality as a "sociopathic personality disturbance," while the *DSM-II* gave homosexuality priority of place as the very first example of its "sexual deviations," described as follows:

> This category is for individuals whose sexual interests are directed primarily toward objects other than people of the opposite sex, toward sexual acts not usually associated with coitus, or toward coitus performed under bizarre circumstances. Even though many find their practices distasteful, they remain unable to substitute normal sexual behavior for them.

One leading proponent of the homosexuality diagnosis was psychiatrist Charles Socarides, a prominent member of the Columbia University Center for Psychoanalytic Training and Research. He believed that homosexuality was not a choice, crime, or immoral act—it was a form of neurosis that originated with "smothering mothers and abdicating fathers." Thus, Socarides argued, homosexuality could be treated like any other neurotic conflict. From the mid-1950s through the mid-1990s, he attempted to "cure" gay men by trying to help them unearth childhood conflicts and thereby convert their sexual orientation to heterosexuality. There's precious little evidence, however, that anyone was ever "cured" of homosexuality through psychoanalysis (or any other therapy, for that matter).

It often happens that one's personal theories of mental illness are put to the test when a family member comes down with the illness, such as when R. D. Laing's theory of schizophrenia as a symbolic journey was challenged after his own daughter became schizophrenic. (Laing ultimately discarded his theory.) Charles Socarides's son Richard was born the same year that he began treating homosexual patients, and as an adolescent he came out as gay, denouncing his father's ideas. Richard went on to become the highest-ranking openly gay man to serve in the federal government, as an advisor to President Clinton. Unlike Laing, Socarides remained unwavering in his conviction that homosexuality was an illness until the end of his life.

Homosexuals viewed their condition quite differently than psychiatrists did. In the late 1960s, many gay men felt empowered by the tremendous social activism going on around them—peace rallies, civil rights marches, abortion law protests, feminist sit-ins. They began to form their own activist groups (such as the Gay Liberation Front) and hold their own demonstrations (such as Gay Pride protests against sodomy laws that criminalized gay sex) that challenged society's blindered perceptions of homosexuality. Not surprisingly, one of the most visible and compelling targets for the early gay rights movement was psychiatry.

Gay men began to speak publicly about their painful experiences in therapy, especially during psychoanalysis. Inspired by psychiatry's rosy promises of becoming "weller than well," gay men sought out shrinks in order to feel better about them-

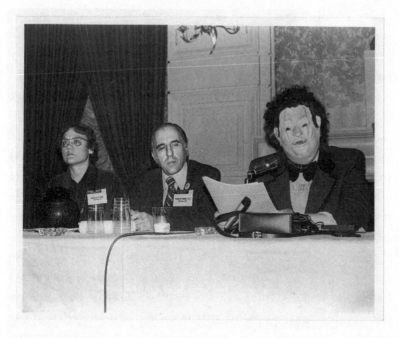

John Fryer in disguise as "Dr. H. Anonymous," with Barbara Gittings and Frank Kameny, at a 1972 APA conference on homosexuality and mental illness entitled "Psychiatry: Friend or Foe to Homosexuals? A Dialogue." (Kay Tobin/©Manuscripts and Archives Division, New York Public Library)

selves, but ended up feeling even more unworthy and unwanted. Especially harrowing were the all too common stories of psychiatrists attempting to reshape homosexuals' sexual identity using hypnosis, confrontational methods, and even aversion therapies that delivered painful electrical shocks to a man's body—sometimes targeting his genitals.

In 1970, gay rights groups demonstrated at the APA annual meeting in San Francisco for the first time, joining forces with the burgeoning antipsychiatry movement. Gay activists formed a human chain around the convention center and blocked psychiatrists from entering the meeting. In 1972, the New York Gay Alliance decided to "zap" a meeting of behavior therapists, using a rudimentary form of a flash mob to call for the end of aversion techniques. Also in 1972, a psychiatrist and gay rights activist named John Fryer delivered a speech at the APA annual meeting under the name Dr. H. Anonymous. He wore a tuxedo, wig, and fright mask that concealed his face while speaking through a special microphone that distorted his voice. His famous speech started with the words, "I am a homosexual. I am a psychiatrist." He went on to describe the oppressive lives of gay psychiatrists who felt compelled to hide their sexual orientation from their colleagues for fear of discrimination while simultaneously hiding their profession from other gay men due to the gay community's disdain for psychiatry.

Robert Spitzer was impressed by the energy and candor of the gay activists. He did not know any gay friends or colleagues before he was assigned to deal with the controversy and suspected that homosexuality probably merited classification as a mental disorder. But the passion of the activists convinced him that the issue should be discussed openly and ultimately settled through data and thoughtful debate.

He organized a panel at the next annual APA meeting, in Honolulu, on the question of whether homosexuality should be a diagnosis in the *DSM*. The panel featured a debate between psychiatrists who were convinced that homosexuality resulted from a flawed upbringing and psychiatrists who believed there was no meaningful evidence to suggest homosexuality was a mental illness. At Spitzer's invitation, Ronald Gold, a member of the Gay Alliance and an influential gay liberationist, was also given the opportunity to express his views on the legitimacy of homosexuality as a psychiatric diagnosis. The event drew an audience of more than a thousand mental health professionals and gay men and women and was heavily covered by the press. Afterward, it was widely reported that the anti-illness proponents had carried the day.

A few months later, Gold brought Spitzer to a secret meeting of a group of gay psychiatrists. Spitzer was stunned to discover that several of the attendees were chairs of prominent psychiatry departments and that another was a former APA president, all living double lives. When they first noticed Spitzer's unexpected presence, they were surprised and outraged, viewing him as a member of the APA establishment who would likely out them, destroying their careers and family relationships. Gold reassured them that Spitzer could be trusted and was their best hope for a fair and thorough review of whether homosexuality should remain in the *DSM*.

After talking with the attendees, Spitzer was persuaded that there was no credible data indicating that being homosexual was the result of any pathologic process or impaired one's mental functioning. "All these gay activists were really nice guys, so friendly, attentive, and compassionate. It became clear to me that being homosexual didn't impair one's ability to effectively function in society at a high level," he explains. By the meeting's end, he felt convinced that diagnosis 302.0, homosexuality, should be eliminated from the *DSM-II*.

But Spitzer found himself in a troubling intellectual bind. On one hand, the antipsychiatry movement was stridently arguing that all mental illnesses were artificial social constructions perpetuated by power-hungry psychiatrists. Like everyone at the APA, Spitzer knew these arguments were taking a toll on the credibility of his profession. He believed that mental illnesses were genuine medical disorders rather than social constructs—but now he was about to declare homosexuality to be exactly such a social construct. If he disavowed homosexuality, he could open the door to the antipsychiatrists to argue that other disorders, such as schizophrenia and depression, should also be disavowed. Even more worrying, perhaps insurance companies would use the decision to rescind the diagnosis of homosexuality as a pretext to stop paying for *any* psychiatric treatments.

On the other hand, if Spitzer maintained that homosexuality was a medical disorder in order to preserve psychiatry's credibility, he now realized that it would cause immeasurable harm to healthy men and women who just happened to be attracted to members of their own sex. Psychoanalysis offered no way out of this bind, since its practitioners' staunch position was that homosexuality arose from traumatic conflicts in childhood. Spitzer finally resolved the conundrum by inventing a new psychiatric concept, a concept that would soon prove pivotal in the next, groundbreaking edition of the *DSM*: *subjective distress.*

Spitzer began to argue that if there was no clear evidence that a patient's condition caused him emotional distress or impaired his ability to function, and if a patient insisted he was well, then a label of illness should not be imposed. If someone claimed that she was content, comfortable, and functioning adequately, then who was the psychiatrist to say otherwise? (According to Spitzer's line of reasoning, even if a schizophrenic insisted he was well, the fact that he was unable to maintain relationships or a job would justify the label of illness.) By endorsing the principle of subjective distress, Spitzer made it plain that homosexuality was not a mental disorder and on its own did not warrant any kind of psychiatric intervention.

This view still allowed for the possibility that if a gay person *asked* for help, insisting he was experiencing anxiety or depression as a direct result of being gay, then psychiatry could still intervene. Spitzer suggested such cases should be considered as a new diagnosis of "sexual orientation disturbance," an approach that left open the possibility of psychiatrists attempting to change the orientation of someone who *asked* psychiatrists to do so. (Spitzer eventually came to regret endorsing any form of sexual orientation conversion.)

When Spitzer's proposal reached the APA Council on

Research to which the Committee on Nomenclature and Assessment reported, it voted unanimously to approve the deletion of the diagnosis of homosexuality disorder from the *DSM-II* and to replace it with the more limited diagnosis of sexual orientation disturbance. On December 15, 1973, the APA Board of Trustees accepted the council's recommendation, and the change was officially incorporated as a revision to the *DSM-II.*

Spitzer expected that this would evoke an uproar from within psychiatry, but instead his colleagues praised him for forging a creative compromise that was humane and practical: a solution that forestalled the antipsychiatrists and simultaneously announced to the world that homosexuality was not an illness. "The irony was that after all was said and done," recalls Spitzer, "the strongest criticism that I received was from those at my home institution, the Columbia Psychoanalytic Center."

In 1987, sexual orientation disturbance was also eliminated as a disorder from the *DSM*. In 2003, the APA established the John E. Fryer Award in honor of Fryer's masked speech as Dr. Anonymous. The award is given annually to a public figure who has made significant contributions to lesbian, gay, bisexual, and transgender (LGBT) mental health. Then in 2013, Dr. Saul Levin became the first openly gay leader of the American Psychiatric Association when he was appointed chief executive officer and medical director.

While American psychiatry was disgracefully slow in eliminating homosexuality as a mental illness, the rest of the world has been even slower. The International Classification of Disease published by the World Health Organization did not eliminate "Homosexuality Disorder" until 1990 and to this very day still lists "Sexual Orientation Disturbance" as a diagnostic condition. This prejudicial diagnosis is often cited by countries that pass antihomosexuality laws, such as Russia and Nigeria.

However, the media did not treat the 1973 elimination of homosexuality disorder from the Bible of Psychiatry as a progressive triumph for psychiatry. Instead, newspapers and antipsychiatrists mocked the APA for "deciding mental illness by democratic vote." Either a mental illness was a medical condition or it wasn't, these critics jeered—you wouldn't find neurologists voting to decide whether a blocked blood vessel in the brain was actually a stroke, would you? Instead of providing a much-needed boost to its public image, the episode proved to be another embarrassment for the beleaguered profession.

Despite the fact that the rest of the world didn't see it that way, Spitzer had managed to orchestrate an impressive feat of diagnostic diplomacy. He had introduced an influential new way of thinking about mental illness in terms of subjective distress, satisfied the gay activists, and effectively parried the antipsychiatry critics. These feats were not lost on the leaders of the American Psychiatric Association.

When the APA Board of Trustees met in the emergency special policy meeting at the peak of the antipsychiatry crisis in February of 1973, they realized that the best way to deflect the tidal wave of reproof was to produce a fundamental change in the way that mental illness was conceptualized and diagnosed—a change rooted in empirical science rather than Freudian dogma. The leaders agreed that the most compelling means for demonstrating this change was by transforming the APA's official compendium of mental illness.

By the end of the emergency meeting, the trustees had authorized the creation of the third edition of the *Diagnostic and Statistical Manual* and instructed the forthcoming *DSM* Task Force "to define Mental Illness and define What is a Psychiatrist." But if the APA wanted to move beyond Freudian theory—a theory that still dictated how the vast majority of psychiatrists diagnosed their patients—then how on earth should mental illness be defined?

One psychiatrist had the answer. "As soon as the special policy meeting voted to authorize a new *DSM*, I knew I wanted

to be in charge." Spitzer recalls. "I spoke to the medical director at the APA and told him I would love to head this thing."
Knowing that the new edition of the *DSM* would require radical changes, and observing how adroitly Spitzer handled the
contentious quandary over homosexuality, the APA Board
appointed Spitzer to chair the *DSM-III* Task Force.

Spitzer knew if he wanted to change the way psychiatry
diagnosed patients, he would need an entirely new system for
defining mental illness—a system rooted in observation and
data rather than tradition and dogma. But in 1973, there was
only one place in the entire United States that had ever developed such a system.

The Feighner Criteria

In the 1920s, the sparse contingent of American psychoanalysts felt lonely and ignored, tucked away on their own little
psychiatric island apart from a continent of alienists. But by
the time of the 1973 emergency session of the APA, the tables
had turned. Psychoanalysts had managed to recast the entire
body of American psychiatry in Freud's image, causing the few
surviving biological and Kraepelinian psychiatrists to feel isolated and beleaguered.

Only a handful of institutions had managed to resist the
psychoanalytic invasion and maintain a balanced approach
to psychiatric research. The most notable of these rare hold-
outs was appropriately located in the "Show-Me" State of
Missouri. Three psychiatrists at Washington University in St.
Louis—Eli Robins, Samuel Guze, and George Winokur—
broke from their colleagues in academic psychiatry by taking a
very different approach to diagnosis. They rested their iconoclastic sensibilities upon one indisputable fact: Nobody had
ever demonstrated that unconscious conflicts (or anything

else) actually caused mental illness. Without clear proof of a causal relationship, Robins, Guze, and Winokur insisted that diagnoses should not be contrived out of mere inference and speculation. The Freudians might have convinced themselves of the existence of neurosis, but it was not a scientific diagnosis. But if medicine lacked any concrete knowledge of what caused the various mental illnesses, then how did the Washington University trio believe they should be defined? By resurrecting the approach of Emil Kraepelin focused on symptoms and their course.

If a specific set of symptoms and their temporal course for each putative disorder could be agreed upon, then each physician would diagnose illnesses in the same way, no matter what her training background or theoretical orientation. This would finally ensure consistency and reliability in diagnosis, asserted the Washington University group—qualities that were egregiously absent in the *DSM-I* and *II*. The trio believed Kraepelin could save psychiatry.

Robins, Guze, and Winokur all came from eastern European families that had recently immigrated to the United States. They ate lunch together every day, brainstorming ideas, united by a sense of common purpose and by their isolation from the rest of psychiatry. (Their outcast status meant that the NIMH denied them funding for clinical studies from the 1950s until the late 1960s.) According to Guze, in the 1960s the Washington University psychiatrists gradually began to realize, "There were people around the country who wanted something different in psychiatry and were looking for someone or some place to take the lead. For many years that was a big advantage to us when it came to recruitment. Residents who were looking for something other than psychoanalytic training were always told to go out to St. Louis. We got a lot of interesting residents." One of these interesting residents was John Feighner.

After graduating from medical school at the University of Kansas, Feighner initially planned to train in internal medicine, but he was drafted into military service. He served as an army physician caring for Vietnam veterans. The experience left him so shaken by the psychic devastation of the soldiers he treated that after he was discharged, he changed direction, and in 1966 he went to Washington University for training in psychiatry.

In his third year as a resident, Feighner was invited to attend meetings with Robins, Guze, and Winokur. He quickly absorbed their Kraepelinian perspective on diagnosis and decided to try to develop diagnostic criteria for depression based upon their ideas. He reviewed close to a thousand published articles about mood disorders and proposed specific symptoms for depression based upon the data in these papers. Impressed with their resident's swift progress, the Washington University trinity formed a committee to help Feighner—and encouraged him to find criteria not just for depression but for all known mental illnesses.

The committee, which also included Washington University psychiatrists Robert Woodruff and Rod Munoz, met every week or two over a period of nine months. Feighner worked tirelessly, bringing every possible paper he could find on every disorder to the committee for review and using this research to propose criteria that were debated, refined, and endorsed by the group. In 1972, Feighner published their final system in the prestigious *Archives of General Psychiatry* as "Diagnostic criteria for use in psychiatric research," though his system soon became immortalized as the Feighner Criteria. The paper concluded with a deliberate shot across the bow of psychoanalysis: "These symptoms represent a synthesis based on data, rather than opinion or tradition."

The Feighner Criteria eventually became one of the most influential publications in the history of medicine and one of the most cited papers ever published in a psychiatric journal, receiving an average of 145 citations per year from the time of its publication through 1980; in contrast, the average article published in the *Archives of General Psychiatry* during the same period received only two citations per year. But when Feighner's paper was first published, it had almost no meaningful impact on clinical practice. To most psychiatrists, the Washington University diagnostic system seemed like a pointless academic exercise, an esoteric research instrument with little relevance to treating the neurotics they saw in their clinical work. But a few psychiatrists did take notice. One was Robert Spitzer. Another was me.

Five years after the publication of his paper, John Feighner came to St. Vincent's Hospital in New York where I was a second-year resident and gave a talk about his new diagnostic criteria. Feighner was physically unimpressive, but his brash manner and energetic intelligence made for a charismatic presence. His ideas resonated with my own growing disenchantment with psychoanalysis and spoke to the confusing clinical reality I was facing with my patients every day.

As was the custom, the St. Vincent's residents had lunch with the speaker following his lecture. Over pizza and soda, we peppered Feighner with questions, and I recall being an over-eager interrogator; I even followed him out of the building and all the way down the street while he hailed a taxi so I could continue talking to him as long as possible. He told me he had just moved to join the faculty of the newly established psychiatry department at the University of California in San Diego and opened a private psychiatric hospital in nearby Rancho Santa Fe that employed his new diagnostic methods, the first of its kind. This encounter with Feighner proved quite fortuitous for me.

A few months after I met Feighner, I received a call from an uncle who informed me that his daughter, my cousin Catherine, was having problems while attending a midwestern college. I was surprised, since I had grown up with her and knew her as intelligent, sensible, and grounded. But according to her father, she was out of control. She stayed out late partying, getting drunk, having risky sex, and engaging in numerous tumultuous relationships. But she would also tuck herself away in her room for days at a time, skipping classes and refusing to see anyone. My uncle didn't know what to do.

I called Cathy's roommate and the resident counselor in her dorm. From their concerned descriptions it seemed that she was probably suffering from some form of manic-depressive illness, today called bipolar disorder. Though her university offered mental health services, the staff consisted of psychologists and social workers who mainly provided counseling. The psychiatry department at the university, meanwhile, was run by psychoanalysts, as were all of the eminent psychiatric centers at the time (including the Menninger Clinic, Austen Riggs, Chestnut Lodge, Sheppard Pratt, and the Payne Whitney Clinic). I had begun to question the effectiveness of psychoanalytical treatments, and didn't want to consign my cousin to misguided care at any of these Freudian institutions. But, then, how to help Cathy? An inspired idea suddenly occurred to me: I would call John Feighner.

I explained Cathy's situation and worked out a plan for her admission to his new hospital halfway across the country, arranging for her to be directly under his care. Following her arrival, Feighner confirmed my provisional diagnosis of manic-depressive illness using his Feighner Criteria, treated her with lithium (a new and highly controversial drug), and within weeks had stabilized her condition. Cathy was discharged, resumed her classes, and graduated on time.

Today I argue against sending patients out of state for psychiatric treatment, since it's usually possible to find competent care locally. But in 1977, at that early stage in my career, I did not have sufficient confidence in my own profession to risk the health of someone dear to me to psychiatry's existing standard of care.

While Feighner made a big impression on me, his criteria were mostly greeted with yawns. According to historian Hannah Decker, the Kraepelinians at Washington University were not surprised by their lack of impact, believing they would be "lucky" to make "a dent" in a field ruled by psychoanalysis.

They turned out to be very lucky indeed.

A Book That Changed Everything

"The Washington University people were absolutely delighted I got the job because they were completely outside of the mainstream, but now I was going to use their diagnostic system for the *DSM*," Spitzer says, smiling. Spitzer had been introduced to the Washington University group in 1971, two years before he was appointed chair of the *DSM-III*, while working on an NIMH study of depression. The head of the project suggested that Spitzer visit Washington University to check out the Kraepelin-influenced ideas about diagnosing depression that originated with Feighner and the Robins, Guze, Winokur triad. "When I got there and discovered they were actually establishing menus of symptoms for each disorder based on data from published research," Spitzer recounts with obvious pleasure, "it was like I had finally awoken from a spell. Finally, a rational way to approach diagnosis other than the nebulous psychoanalytical definitions in the *DSM-II.*"

Armed with the Feighner Criteria and determined to counteract the claims of the antipsychiatry movement by establishing rock-solid reliability in diagnosis, Spitzer's first job as chairman was to appoint the other members of the *DSM-III* Task Force. "Outside of the APA Board, nobody really cared much about the new *DSM*, so it was totally under my control," Spitzer explains. "I didn't have to clear my appointments with anyone—so about half my appointees were Feighner types."

When the seven Task Force members assembled for the first time, each expected to be the odd person out, believing their desire for increased objectivity and precision in diagnosis would represent the minority view. To their surprise, they discovered that, as a group, they unanimously favored the "dust bowl empiricism" of Washington University: There was universal consensus that the *DSM-II* should be unabashedly jettisoned, while the *DSM-III* should use specifically defined, symptoms-based criteria instead of general descriptions. Task Force member Nancy Andreasen of the University of Iowa recalls, "We shared the feeling we were creating a small revolution in American psychiatry."

Spitzer established twenty-five separate *DSM-III* subcommittees, each asked to produce detailed descriptions for one domain of mental illness, such as anxiety disorders, mood disorders, or sexual disorders. To fill these committees, Spitzer appointed psychiatrists who saw themselves primarily as scientists rather than clinicians and instructed them to scour published data relative to the establishment of possible diagnostic criteria—regardless of whether these data-based criteria aligned with the traditional understanding of a disorder.

Spitzer threw himself into the creation of a new *DSM* with a fierce and focused energy. "I was working seven days a week, sometimes twelve hours a day," he recollects. "Sometimes I would wake up Janet in the middle of the night asking for her opinion on a point, and then she'd get up and we'd work together." Spitzer's wife, Janet Williams, who has a doctorate in social work and is a leading expert in diagnostic assessment, confirms that the *DSM-III* was an all-consuming project for them both. "He answered every letter the Task Force received while he was working on the *DSM-III*, and responded to every critical article about it, no matter how obscure the journal—and remember, this was before computers," Janet recounts. "Fortunately, we were very fast typists." Jean Endicott, a psychologist who worked closely with Spitzer, remembers, "He would come in on Mondays having clearly worked on the *DSM* all weekend. If you sat by him on the plane, there was no question what you were going to be talking about."

Spitzer soon proposed an idea that—if adopted—would fundamentally and irrevocably alter the medical definition of mental illness. He suggested dropping the one criterion that psychoanalysts had long considered essential when diagnosing a patient's illness: the *cause* of the illness, or what physicians term *etiology*. Ever since Freud, psychoanalysts believed that mental illness was caused by unconscious conflicts. Identify the conflicts and you would identify the illness, ran the venerable Freudian doctrine. Spitzer rejected this approach. He shared the Washington University group's view that there was no evidence to support the cause of *any* mental illness (other than addictions). He wanted to expunge all references to etiology that weren't backed up by hard data. The rest of the Task Force unanimously agreed.

To replace causes, Spitzer laid down two new essential criteria for any diagnosis: (1) the symptoms must be distressing to the individual *or* the symptoms must impair the individual's ability to function (this was the "subjective distress" criteria he had first proposed while fighting to depathologize homosexuality), and (2) the symptoms must be enduring (so if you were gloomy for a day after your pet hamster died, this would not constitute depression).

This was a definition of mental illness radically different from anything before. Not only was it far removed from the psychoanalytical view that a patient's mental illness could be hidden from the patient herself, but it also amended Emil

Kraepelin's definition, which made no reference to subjective distress and considered short-lived conditions to be illnesses, too.

Spitzer laid down a two-step process for diagnosing patients that was as simple as it was shockingly new: first, determine the presence (or absence) of specific symptoms and for how long they had been active; then, compare these observed symptoms to the fixed set of criteria for each disorder. If the symptoms matched the criteria, then a diagnosis was justified. That's it. No ferreting around in a patient's unconscious for clues to a diagnosis, no interpreting the latent symbolism of dreams — just identifying concrete behaviors, thoughts, and physiological manifestations.

The *DSM-III* Task Force learned very quickly that in order to remain faithful to the published data, it was often necessary to create rather complex sets of criteria. In the *DSM-II*, for example, schizophrenia was dealt with in a series of impressionistic descriptions, including this definition of paranoid schizophrenia:

> This type of schizophrenia is characterized primarily by the presence of persecutory or grandiose delusions, often associated with hallucinations. Excessive religiosity is sometimes seen. The patient's attitude is frequently hostile and aggressive, and his behavior tends to be consistent with the delusions.

By contrast, the *DSM-III* provided several sets and subsets of conditions that were required for a diagnosis of schizophrenia. Here, for example, is condition C:

> C. At least three of the following manifestations must be present for a diagnosis of "definite" schizophrenia, and two for a diagnosis of "probable" schizophrenia. (1) Single.

(2) Poor premorbid social adjustment or work history. (3) Family history of schizophrenia. (4) Absence of alcoholism or drug abuse within one year of onset of psychosis. (5) Onset of illness prior to age 40.

Critics quickly sneered at the complicated "Select one from criteria set A, select two from criteria set B" instructions, calling it the "Chinese menu" approach to diagnosis, after the multitiered menus that were common in Chinese restaurants at the time. Spitzer and the Task Force countered that this increased complexity in the diagnostic criteria matched the evidence-based reality of mental disorders far better than the ambiguous generalities of the *DSM-II.*

But there was one notable problem with the Task Force's utopian vision of better psychiatry through science: For many disorders, the science hadn't actually been done yet. How could Spitzer determine which symptoms constituted a disorder when so few psychiatrists outside of Washington University and a handful of other institutions were conducting rigorous research on symptoms? What the Task Force needed were cross-sectional and longitudinal studies of patients' symptoms and how these patterns of symptoms persisted over time, how they ran in families, how they responded to treatment, and how they reacted to life events. While Spitzer insisted that the diagnoses be based on published data, such data were often in very short supply.

If there was not an extensive body of literature on a particular diagnosis, then the Task Force followed an orderly procedure. First they reached out to researchers for unpublished data or gray literature (technical reports, white papers, or other research not published in a peer-reviewed format). Next, they reached out to experts with experience with the tentative diagnosis. Finally, the entire Task Force would debate the putative criteria until they reached consensus. Spitzer told me, "We tried to make the criteria represent the best thinking of people who had the most expertise in the area. The guiding principle was that the criteria needed to be logical and rational." The *DSM-III* added many new disorders, including attention-deficit disorder, autism, anorexia nervosa, bulimia, panic disorder, and post-traumatic stress disorder.

There was one overt nonscientific factor that influenced the new diagnostic criteria: ensuring that insurance companies would pay for treatments. Spitzer knew that insurance companies were already cutting back on mental health care benefits as a result of the antipsychiatry movement. To combat this, the *DSM-III* stressed that its criteria were not the ultimate diagnostic word but that "clinical judgment is of paramount importance in making a diagnosis." They believed that this disclaimer would give psychiatrists protection against an insurance company intent on showing that a patient did not exactly conform to the criteria listed. In actuality, time has shown that insurance companies do not tend to challenge psychiatrists' diagnoses—instead, they often challenge the choice and duration of *treatment* for a diagnosis.

The *DSM-III* represented a revolutionary approach to mental illness, neither psychodynamic nor biological, but able to incorporate new research from any theoretical camp. By rejecting causes (including neurosis) as diagnostic criteria, the *DSM-III* also represented a complete repudiation of psychoanalytic theory. Before the *DSM-III*, the Feighner Criteria had almost exclusively been used for academic research, rather than clinical practice. Now the *DSM-III* would render the Feighner Criteria the clinical law of the land. But first, there was one major hurdle to surmount, and it was a doozy.

The *DSM-III* would only be published by the APA if its members voted to approve it. In 1979, a strong and vocal majority of these members were psychoanalysts. How could Spitzer persuade them to endorse a book that ran counter to their approach and might spell their own doom?

The Showdown

Throughout his tenure, Spitzer transparently and continuously communicated the Task Force's progress on the *DSM-III* via a steady stream of personal letters, meeting minutes, reports, bulletins, publications, and talks. Each time he made a public presentation or published an update on the *DSM-III*, he encountered pushback. At first, the criticism was relatively mild, since most psychiatrists had no vested interest in a new diagnostic manual. Gradually, as more and more was revealed about the contents of the *DSM-III*, the blowback intensified.

The turning point came in June 1976 at a special meeting in St. Louis (sponsored by the University of Missouri, not Washington University) with an audience of one hundred leaders in psychiatry and psychology. The *DSM-III* in Midstream, as the conference was called, marked the first time that many prominent psychoanalysts heard about Spitzer's new vision for diagnosis. This was when the cat was finally let out of the bag. The meeting exploded in controversy. Attendees denounced what they viewed as a sterile system that purged the *DSM* of its intellectual substance, claiming Spitzer was turning the art of diagnosis into a mechanical exercise. Spitzer was frequently accosted in the corridors by psychoanalysts who demanded to know if he was intentionally setting out to destroy psychiatry, and by psychologists who demanded to know if he was deliberately attempting to marginalize their profession.

When it was over, influential groups mobilized to oppose Spitzer; he responded by throwing himself with redoubled energy into the task of responding to the opposition. Two of the most formidable opponents were the American Psychological Association, the largest professional organization of psychologists (sometimes referred to as "the big APA" since there are far more psychologists than psychiatrists in the U.S.), and the

American Psychoanalytic Association (APsaA), still the largest professional organization of Freudian psychiatrists. One of the original goals of the *DSM-III* was to firmly establish that mental illness was a genuine medical condition in order to push back against the antipsychiatry movement's contention that mental illness was merely a cultural label. But psychologists—therapists with a PhD instead of an MD—had benefited greatly from the antipsychiatry argument. If mental illness was a social phenomenon, as Szasz, Goffman, and Laing charged, then one didn't need a medical degree to treat it: Anyone could justifiably use psychotherapy to guide a patient through her problems. If the American Psychiatric Association formally declared that mental illness was a medical disorder, psychologists stood to have their recent professional gains rolled back.

At first, the president of the big APA, Charles Kiesler, wrote to the American Psychiatric Association in diplomatic fashion: "I do not wish partisan conflict between our associations. In that spirit, the American Psychological Association wishes to offer its complete services to assist the American Psychiatric Association in the further development of the *DSM-III*." Spitzer's response was equally cordial: "We certainly believe that the American Psychological Association is in a unique position to help us in our work." He included, with his reply, the latest draft of the *DSM-III*—which unambiguously asserted that mental illness was a medical condition. Now President Kiesler cut to the chase:

> Since there is an implication that mental disorders are diseases, this suggests that social workers, psychologists, and educators lack the training and skills to diagnose, treat, or manage such disorders. If the current approach is not altered, then the American Psychological Association will embark on its own truly empirical venture in classification of behavioral disorders.

Kiesler's thinly veiled threat to publish his own (nonmedical) version of the *DSM* had an effect other than the one intended: It provided Spitzer with an opening to retain his medical definition. Spitzer wrote back and politely encouraged him and the American Psychological Association to pursue their own classification system, suggesting that such a book might be a valuable contribution to mental health. In reality, Spitzer guessed (correctly) that the formidable demands of pursuing such an undertaking—which he was in the midst of himself—would ultimately prevent the big APA from pulling it off; at the same time, his endorsement of Kiesler's project provided Spitzer with cover for the *DSM-III*'s medical definition— after all, the psychologists were free to put their own definition of mental illness in their own book.

But Spitzer's biggest battle by far—truly a battle for the soul of psychiatry—was a winner-take-all clash with the psychoanalysts. Psychoanalytic institutions did not pay much attention to the *DSM-III* Task Force for the first two years of its existence, and not just because they didn't care about the classification of mental disorders. They simply had little to fear from anyone: For four decades, the Freudians had ruled the profession unchecked. They controlled the academic departments, university hospitals, private practices, and even (so they assumed) the American Psychiatric Association; they were the face, voice, and pocketbook of psychiatry. It was simply inconceivable that something as insignificant as a classification manual would threaten their supreme authority. As Donald Klein, a member of the *DSM-III* Task Force, put it, "For the psychoanalysts, to be interested in descriptive diagnosis was to be superficial and a little bit stupid."

The Midstream conference had roused the psychoanalysts from their apathy, though, forcing them to confront the possible effects of the *DSM-III* on the practice and public perception of psychoanalysis. Shortly after the conference, one prominent psychoanalyst wrote to Spitzer, "The *DSM-III* gets rid of the castle of neurosis and replaces it with a diagnostic Levittown," comparing Spitzer's *Manual* to a cookie-cutter housing development being built on Long Island. Two other prominent psychoanalysts charged that "the elimination of the psychiatric past by the *DSM-III* Task Force can be compared to the director of a national museum destroying his Rembrandts, Goyas, Utrillos, van Goghs, etc. because he believes his collection of Comic-Strip Type Warhols has greater relevance."

But on the whole, since the psychoanalysts still had such a hard time believing that anything meaningful would come out of Spitzer's project, there was never any great urgency behind their response. After all, the publication of the *DSM-I* and *DSM-II* had produced no noticeable impact on their profession. It took more than nine months after the Midstream conference for the first group of psychoanalysts to approach Spitzer with a formal request. The president and president-elect of the American Psychoanalytic Association sent a telegram to the APA asking that they postpone any more work on the *DMS-III* until the American Psychoanalytic Association had a chance to thoroughly evaluate its existing content and review the process by which any additional content would be approved. The APA refused.

In September of 1977, a liaison committee was formed consisting of four or five psychoanalysts from the APsaA who began to pepper Spitzer and the Task Force with requests. At about the same time, another group of four or five psychoanalysts from the powerful Washington, DC, branch of the APA also began to lobby for changes in the *DSM-III*. The Washington branch was probably the most influential and best organized unit of the APA, owing to the large number of psychiatrists in the nation's capital drawing business from the superior mental health benefits offered to federal employees. For the next six months, Spitzer and the psychoanalysts jousted over changes to the definitions of disorders.

At one point, Spitzer informed the Task Force that he was going to concede to some of the psychoanalysts' requests as a political necessity to ensure the adoption of the *DSM-III*. To his surprise, the other Task Force members unanimously voted him down. Spitzer had chosen his Task Force because of their commitment to sweeping changes, and now their uncompromising devotion to these principles exceeded his own. Emboldened by his own team to hold the line, Spitzer repeatedly informed the psychoanalysts that he could not fulfill their requests.

As the critical vote drew near, psychoanalytic factions presented alternative proposals and engaged in frenzied efforts to pressure Spitzer into accepting their demands. But Spitzer, having devoted almost every waking hour to the *DSM* for four years, was always ready with a response that drew upon scientific evidence and practical arguments to support his position, while the psychoanalysts were often left stammering that Freudian psychoanalysis needed to be upheld on the basis of history and tradition. "There were disputes over the placement of each word, the use of modifiers, the capitalization of entries," Spitzer told historian Hannah Decker. "Each adjustment, each attempt at fine tuning, carried with it symbolic importance to those engaged in a process that was at once political and scientific."

Spitzer plowed through the testy negotiations and contentious wordsmithing until he had a final draft in early 1979. All that remained was for it to be ratified at the May meeting of the APA Assembly. With the vote looming, the psychoanalysts finally appreciated just how high the stakes were and ratcheted up the pressure on both the Task Force and the APA Board of

Trustees with fierce determination, frequently warning that the psychoanalysts would abandon the *DSM-III* (and the APA) en masse if their demands were not met. As the long-awaited date of the vote approached, the final counterassault launched by Spitzer's opponents targeted a critical component of psychoanalysis—*neurosis*. Neurosis was the fundamental concept of psychoanalytic theory and represented to its practitioners the very definition of mental illness. It was also the primary source of professional revenue in clinical practice, since the idea that *everyone* suffers from some kind of neurotic conflict drove a steady stream of the worried well onto shrinks' couches. As you can imagine, the psychoanalysts were horrified when they learned that Spitzer intended to expunge neurosis from psychiatry.

The influential and iconoclastic psychiatrist Roger Peele was the head of the DC branch of the APA at the time. While Peele generally supported Spitzer's diagnostic vision, he felt obligated to challenge Spitzer on behalf of his psychoanalytic constituency. "The most common diagnosis in DC in the 1970s was something called depressive neurosis," Peele said. "That was what they were doing day after day." He put forward a compromise plan called the Peele Proposal, which argued for the inclusion of a neurosis diagnosis "to avoid an unnecessary break with the past." The Task Force shot it down.

In the final days before the vote, a flurry of other proposals were put forth to save neurosis, with names like the Talbott Plan, the Burris Modification, the McGrath initiative, and Spitzer's own Neurotic Peace Plan. All were rejected by one side or the other. At last, the fateful morning arrived—May 12, 1979. Even at this late stage, the psychoanalysts made one final push. Spitzer countered with a compromise: While the *DSM* would not include any neurosis-specific diagnoses, it would list alternative psychoanalytical names for certain diagnoses without changing the criteria for the diagnoses (such as "hypochondriacal neurosis" for hypochondriasis or "obsessive-compulsive neurosis" for obsessive-compulsive disorder), and one appendix would include descriptions of "Neurotic Disorders" in language similar to the *DSM-II*. But would this paltry concession satisfy the rank-and-file psychoanalysts of the APA Assembly?

Three hundred and fifty psychiatrists gathered together in a large ballroom in the Chicago Conrad Hilton Hotel. Spitzer stepped onto the two-tiered stage, explained the goals of the Task Force, and briefly reviewed the *DSM* process before presenting the final draft of the *DSM-III* to the assembly, parts of it typed up mere hours before. But the psychoanalysts squeezed in one last Hail Mary.

Psychoanalyst Hector Jaso made the motion that the assembly adopt the draft of the *DSM-III*—with one amendment. "Depressive neurosis" would be inserted as a specific diagnosis. Spitzer retorted that its inclusion would violate the consistency and design of the entire *Manual,* and besides—the existence of depressive neurosis simply wasn't supported by the available data. Jaso's motion was put to an oral vote and was resoundingly defeated.

But was the assembly rejecting a last-second change, or voicing disapproval of the entire *DSM-III* project? At long last, after tens of thousands of man-hours of labor, the product of Spitzer's visionary framework, the *DSM-III,* was put to a vote. The assembly was virtually unanimous in their response: *YES*.

"Then a rather remarkable thing happened," Peele reported in *The New Yorker.* "Something that you don't see in the assembly very often. People stood up and applauded." Shock spread across Spitzer's face. And then: "Bob's eyes got watery. Here was a group that he was afraid would torpedo all his efforts and aspirations, and instead he got a standing ovation."

How did Spitzer manage to triumph over psychiatry's ruling

class? Even though the psychoanalysts vigorously resisted his efforts to eliminate Freudian concepts, for most Freudians the benefits of Spitzer's transformative book outweighed its shortcomings. They were, after all, fully aware of psychiatry's public image problem and the threat posed by the antipsychiatrists. They realized that psychiatry needed a makeover and that this makeover had to be grounded in some form of medical science. Even Spitzer's adversaries recognized that his radical new *Diagnostic Manual* offered a lifeline to the entire field, a chance to restore psychiatry's battered reputation.

The *DSM-III*'s impact was just as dramatic as Spitzer hoped. Psychoanalytic theory was permanently banished from psychiatric diagnosis and psychiatric research, and the role of psychoanalysts in APA leadership was greatly diminished thereafter. The *DSM-III* turned psychiatry away from the task of curing social ills and refocused it on the medical treatment of severe mental illnesses. Spitzer's diagnostic criteria could be used with impressive reliability by any psychiatrist from Wichita to Walla Walla. The Elena Conways and Abigail Abercrombies of the world, neglected for so long, once again assumed center stage in American psychiatry.

There were unintended consequences as well. The *DSM-III* forged an uneasy symbiosis between the *Manual* and insurance companies that would soon come to influence every aspect of American mental health care. Insurance companies would only pay for certain conditions listed in the *DSM*, requiring psychiatrists to shoehorn ever more patients into a limited number of diagnoses to ensure that they would be reimbursed for the care provided. Even though the Task Force intended for the *DSM-III* to be used only by health care professionals, the *Manual*'s anointed diagnoses immediately became the de facto map of mental illness for every sector of society. Insurance companies, schools, universities, research funding agencies, pharmaceutical companies, federal and state legislatures, judicial systems, the military, Medicare, and Medicaid all yearned for consistency in psychiatric diagnoses, and in short order all of these institutions tied policies and funding to the *DSM-III*. Never before in the history of medicine had a single document changed so much and affected so many.

I wasn't at the momentous Chicago meeting when the APA Assembly approved the *DSM-III*, though I had the good fortune of presiding over the last public appearance that Spitzer

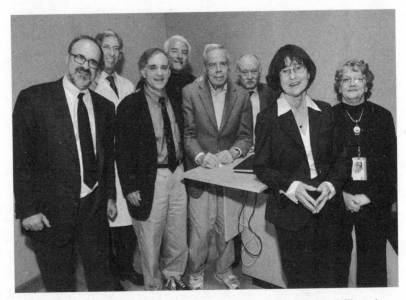

Festschrift for Robert Spitzer. From left to right: Michael First (psychiatrist and protégé of Spitzer who worked on *DSM-III, IV,* and *5*), author Jeffrey Lieberman, Jerry Wakefield (professor of social work at New York University), Allen Frances (psychiatrist, Spitzer protégé, and chair of the *DSM-IV* Task Force), Bob Spitzer (psychiatrist and chair of the *DSM-III* Task Force), Ron Bayer (professor of sociomedical science at Columbia University and author of a book on the removal of homosexuality from the *DSM*), Hannah Dekker (historian and author of *The Making of DSM-III*), and Jean Endicott (psychologist and colleague who worked with Spitzer). (Courtesy of Eve Vagg, New York State Psychiatric Institute)

ever made. Bob was forced into retirement in 2008 by a severe and debilitating form of Parkinson's disease. To mark his retirement, we organized a tribute to celebrate his remarkable achievements that was attended by psychiatric luminaries and Bob's protégés. They took turns speaking about the man who had so profoundly shaped their careers. Finally, Bob rose to speak. He had always been a powerful and disciplined orator, but as he began his remarks he broke into uncontrollable sobs. He was unable to go on, overwhelmed by the sincere show of affection and admiration. As he continued to weep, I gently took the microphone from his trembling hand and told everyone that the last time Bob was speechless at the assembly meeting in Chicago was when the APA passed the *DSM-III*. The audience rose to their feet and gave him an ovation that rolled on and on and on.

Part II

The Story of Treatment

If only his mind were as easy to fix as his body.
— HAN NOLAN

Chapter 5

Desperate Measures: Fever Cures, Coma Therapy, and Lobotomies

What can't be cured must be endured.
— ROBERT BURTON

Rose. Her head cut open.
A knife thrust in her brain.
Me. Here. Smoking.
My father, mean as a
devil, snoring — 1000 miles
away.
— TENNESSEE WILLIAMS, ON HIS
SISTER ROSE'S LOBOTOMY

The Snake Pit

For the first century and a half of psychiatry's existence, the only real treatment for severe mental illness was institutionalization. In 1917, Emil Kraepelin captured the pervasive sense of hopelessness among clinicians when he told his colleagues, "We can rarely alter the course of mental illness. We must openly admit that the vast majority of the patients placed in our institutions are forever lost." Thirty years later, things had hardly improved. The pioneering biological psychiatrist Lothar Kalinowsky wrote in 1947, "Psychiatrists can do little more for patients than make them comfortable, maintain contact with their families, and, in the case of a spontaneous remission, return them to the community." Spontaneous remission — the only ray of hope for the mentally ill from the 1800s through the 1950s—was in most cases about as likely as stumbling upon a four-leaf clover in a snowstorm.

At the start of the nineteenth century, the asylum movement barely existed in the United States, and there were very few institutions dedicated to the mentally ill in which to confine affected individuals. In mid-century the great crusader for the mentally ill, Dorothea Dix, persuaded state legislatures to build mental institutions in significant numbers. By 1904 there were 150,000 patients in asylums, and by 1955, there were more than 550,000. The largest institution was Pilgrim State Hospital, in Brentwood, New York, which at its peak housed 19,000 mental patients on its sprawling campus. The institution was a self-contained city. It possessed its own private water works, electric light plant, heating plant, sewage system, fire department, police department, courts, church, post office, cemetery, laundry, store, amusement hall, athletic fields, greenhouses, and farm.

The ever-expanding number of institutionalized patients was an inescapable reminder of psychiatry's inability to treat severe mental illness. Not surprisingly, when so many incurable patients were forced together, the conditions in asylums often became intolerable. In 1946, a forty-one-year-old writer named Mary Jane Ward published an autobiographical novel, *The Snake Pit*, which depicted her experience in Rockland State Hospital, a mental institution in Orangeburg, New York. After being erroneously diagnosed as schizophrenic, Ward was subjected to an unrelenting stream of horrors that seem the very opposite of therapeutic: rooms overcrowded with unwashed inmates, extended periods in physical restraints, prolonged isolation, raucous noise around the clock, patients wallowing in their own excrement, frigid baths, indifferent attendants.

While the conditions of mental hospitals were undeniably wretched, there was precious little the staff could actually do to improve their patients' lot. The government-supported budgets for state institutions were always inadequate (though they usually ranked among the most expensive items in any state budget), and there were always more patients than the under-funded institutions were built to handle. The bleak reality was that there was simply no effective treatment for the illnesses that afflicted institutionalized patients, so all the asylums could hope to accomplish was try to keep their overcrowded patients warm, well-fed, and free from harm.

When I was in grade school, individuals afflicted with schizo-phrenia, bipolar disorder, major depression, autism, and demen-tia all had little hope for recovery—and virtually no hope at all for stable relationships, gainful employment, or meaningful personal development. Psychiatrists of the era were keenly aware of the abhorrent conditions that their patients experienced inside mental institutions and the overwhelming challenges they faced outside of them, and they longed for something—*anything*—to relieve their patients' suffering. Driven by compas-sion and desperation, asylum-era physicians devised a succession of audacious treatments that today elicit feelings of revulsion or even outrage at their apparent barbarism. Unfortunately, many of these early treatments for mental illness have become forever linked with the public's dismal image of psychiatry.

The simple fact is that the alternative to these crude meth-ods was not some kind of medicinal cure or enlightened psychotherapy—the alternative was interminable misery, as there was nothing that worked. Even the risks of an extreme or danger-ous treatment often seemed worthwhile when weighed against lifelong institutionalization in a place like Pilgrim or Rockland. If we want to fully appreciate just how far psychiatry has progressed—to the point where the vast majority of individuals with severe mental illness have the opportunity to lead a relatively normal and decent life if they receive good treatment instead of wasting away inside the decrepit walls of an asylum—however, we must first confront the desperate measures that psychiatrists pursued in their improbable quest to defeat mental illness.

Fever Cures and Coma Therapy

In the early decades of the twentieth century, asylums were filled with inmates suffering from a peculiar form of psychosis known as "general paresis of the insane," or GPI. It was caused by advanced syphilis. Left untreated, the spiral-shaped micro-organism that caused this venereal disease would burrow into the brain and produce symptoms often indistinguishable from schizophrenia or bipolar disorder. Since syphilis remained untreatable in the early twentieth century, psychiatrists searched frantically for any way to reduce the symptoms experienced by a flood of GPI-demented patients, which included mobster Al Capone and composer Robert Schumann.

In 1917, as Freud was publishing *Introductory Lectures on Psychoanalysis*, another Viennese physician was about to make an equally astonishing discovery. Julius Wagner-Jauregg was the scion of a noble Austrian family. He studied pathology in medical school and then went to work in a psychiatry clinic, where he cared for psychotic patients. One day, he observed something surprising in a GPI patient named Hilda.

Hilda had been lost to the turbulent madness of the disease for more than a year when she came down with a fever entirely unrelated to her syphilis, a symptom of a respiratory infection. When the fever subsided, Hilda awoke clear-headed and lucid. Her psychosis had vanished.

Since the symptoms of GPI typically progressed in only one direction—worse—the remission of Hilda's psychotic symptoms piqued Wagner-Jauregg's interest. What had happened? Since her sanity had been restored immediately after her fever subsided, he surmised that something about the fever itself must be responsible. Perhaps her elevated body temperature had stunned or even killed the syphilis spirochetes in her brain?

Today, we know that fevers are one of the body's oldest and most primitive mechanisms for fighting infection—part of what is known as the "innate immune system." The heat of a fever damages both host and invader, but it is often more damaging to the invader since many pathogens are sensitive to high temperatures. (Our more evolutionarily recent "adaptive immune system" produces the familiar antibodies that target specific invaders.) Lacking any meaningful understanding of the mechanics of fever, Wagner-Jauregg conceived a bold experiment to test the effects of high temperatures on psychosis. How? By infecting GPI patients with fever-producing diseases.

He started out by serving his psychotic patients water containing streptococcal bacteria (the source of strep throat). Next he tried tuberculin, an extract from the bacteria that cause tuberculosis, and eventually malaria, probably because there was a ready supply of malaria-infected blood from soldiers returning from World War I. After Wagner-Jauregg injected his GPI patients with the *Plasmodium* parasites that cause malaria, the patients succumbed to the characteristic fever of malaria...and shortly afterward, exhibited dramatic improvements in their mental state.

Patients who previously behaved bizarrely and talked incoherently now were composed and conversed normally with Dr. Wagner-Jauregg. Some patients even appeared cured of their syphilis entirely. Here in the twenty-first century it may not seem like a favorable bargain to trade one awful disease for another, but at least malaria was treatable with quinine, a cheap and abundant extract of tree bark.

Wagner-Jauregg's new method, dubbed *pyrotherapy*, quickly became the standard treatment for GPI. Even though the idea of intentionally infecting mentally ill patients with malaria parasites raises the hair on the backs of our necks—and indeed, about 15 percent of patients treated with Wagner-Jauregg's fever cure died from the procedure—pyrotherapy represented the very first effective treatment for severe mental illness. Think about that for a moment. Never before in history had *any* medical procedure been shown to alleviate psychosis, the most forbidding and relentless of psychiatric maladies. GPI had always been a one-way ticket to permanent institutionalization or death. Now, those afflicted with the mind-ravaging disease had a reasonable chance of returning to sanity—and possibly returning home. For this stunning achievement, Wagner-Jauregg was awarded the Nobel Prize in Medicine in 1927, the first ever for the field of psychiatry.

Wagner-Jauregg's fever cure instilled hope that there might be other practical ways to treat mental illness. With the benefit of modern hindsight, we might point out that compared to other mental illnesses GPI was highly unusual, since it was caused by an external pathogen infecting the brain. We would hardly expect that a germ-killing procedure would have any effect on other mental illnesses after legions of biological psychiatrists had failed to detect the presence of any foreign agent in patients' brains. Nevertheless, inspired by Wagner-Jauregg's success, many psychiatrists in the 1920s attempted to apply pyrotherapy to other disorders.

In asylums around the country, patients with schizophrenia, depression, mania, and hysteria were soon infected with a wide variety of fever-producing diseases. Some alienists even went so far as to inject malaria-infected blood through the skulls of schizophrenic patients directly into their brains. Alas, pyrotherapy did not turn out to be the panacea that so many had hoped for. Though the fever cure mitigated the psychotic symptoms of GPI, it proved impotent against all other forms of mental illness. Since other disorders were not caused by pathogens, there was nothing for the fever to kill, except, occasionally, the patient.

Even so, the unprecedented effectiveness of pyrotherapy in treating GPI shined the first glimmer of light into the darkness that had dominated asylum psychiatry for over a century. Spurred by Wagner-Jauregg's success, another Austrian psychiatrist, Manfred Sakel, experimented with a physiological technique even more unsettling than malaria therapy. Sakel had been treating drug addicts with low doses of insulin as a way of combatting opiate addiction. Often, heavy users of morphine and opium would exhibit extreme behaviors similar to mental illness, such as relentless pacing, frenetic movement, and disorganized thought. Sakel noticed that when addicts were accidentally given higher doses of insulin, their blood sugar would drop precipitously, inducing a hypoglycemic coma that could last for hours at a time—but after they awoke, they were much calmer, and their extreme behavior had abated. Sakel wondered: Might comas also relieve the symptoms of mental illness?

Sakel began to experiment with artificially induced comas. He overdosed schizophrenic patients with insulin, which had recently been developed as a treatment for diabetes. The insulin overdose put them into a coma, which Sakel ended by administering intravenous glucose. After the patients regained consciousness, Sakel would wait a short while, then repeat the procedure. He would sometimes induce a coma in a patient six days in a row. To his delight, his patients' psychotic symptoms diminished and they showed apparent signs of improvement.

As you might imagine, there were significant risks to Sakel's technique. One side effect was that patients invariably became grossly obese, since insulin pushes glucose into cells. A far more permanent side effect was that a small number of patients never woke from the coma and died outright. The most salient risk was permanent brain damage. The brain consumes a disproportionate share of the body's total glucose (70 percent) despite the fact that it accounts for only 2 percent of the body's weight. Consequently, our organ of consciousness is acutely sensitive to fluctuations in blood glucose levels and easily incurs damage if the levels are low for any stretch of time.

Rather than viewing brain damage as a liability, advocates of Sakel's method claimed it was actually a benefit: If brain damage *did* occur it produced a desirable "loss of tension and hostility," or so Sakel's proponents rationalized.

Like fever therapy, coma therapy became widely adopted by alienists throughout the United States and Europe. It was used at almost every major mental hospital in the 1940s and '50s, with each institution developing its own protocol for administering coma therapy. In some cases, patients were placed into a coma fifty or sixty times during the course of treatment. Despite the manifest risks, psychiatrists marveled at the fact that finally, *finally,* there was something they could do to ease the suffering of their patients, even if temporarily.

Nothing an Ice Pick to the Eye Can't Fix

Ever since the very earliest psychiatrists began conceiving of disturbed behaviors as illnesses (and even long before), they held out hope that direct manipulation of a patient's brain might one day prove therapeutic. In the 1930s, two treatments were developed that promised to fulfill these hopes. One survived a difficult start and a notorious reputation to become a mainstay of contemporary mental health care. The other followed an opposite track, starting out as a promising treatment that was rapidly adopted around the world, but ending up as the most infamous treatment in the history of psychiatry.

Starting many millennia ago with prehistoric cases of trepanation — the drilling of holes through the skull into the brain — physicians have attempted brain surgery as a means of treating the emotional chaos of mental disorder, always without success. In 1933, one Portuguese physician was undeterred by this legacy of failure. António Egas Moniz, a neurologist on the faculty of the University of Lisbon, shared the conviction of the biological psychiatrists that mental illness was a neural condition, and therefore should be treatable through direct intervention in the brain. As a neurologist, he had learned that strokes, tumors, and penetrating brain injuries each impaired behaviors and emotions by damaging a specific part of the brain. He hypothesized that the opposite should also hold true: by damaging an appropriate part of the brain, impaired behaviors and emotions could be rectified. The only question was, what part of the brain should be operated on?

Moniz carefully studied the various regions of the human brain to determine which neural structures might be the most promising candidates for surgery. In particular, he hoped to find the parts of the brain that governed feelings, since he believed that calming a patient's turbulent emotions was the key to treating mental illness. In 1935, Moniz attended a lecture at a medical conference in London where a Yale neurology researcher made an interesting observation: When patients sustained injuries to their frontal lobe, they became emotionally subdued, but, curiously, their ability to think seemed undiminished. Here was the breakthrough Moniz had been looking for—a way to calm the stormy emotions of mental illness while preserving normal cognition.

When he returned to Lisbon, Moniz eagerly set up his first psychosurgery experiment. His target: the frontal lobes. Since Moniz lacked any training in neurosurgery, he recruited a young neurosurgeon, Pedro Almeida Lima, to perform the actual procedure. Moniz's plan was to create lesions—or, to put it more bluntly, inflict permanent brain damage—within the frontal lobes of patients with severe mental disorders, a procedure he dubbed a *leucotomy*.

Moniz performed the first of twenty leucotomies on November 12, 1935, at the Hospital de Santa Marta in Lisbon. Each patient was put to sleep under general anesthesia. Lima drilled two holes in the front of the skull, just above each eye. Then, he performed the crux of the procedure: He inserted the needle of a special syringe-shaped instrument of his own invention—a leucotome—through the hole in the skull. He pressed the plunger on the syringe, which extended a wire loop into the brain. Next, the leucotome was rotated, carving out a small sphere of brain tissue like coring an apple.

How did Moniz and Lima decide where to cut the brain, considering that brain imaging and the use of stereotactic procedures was still far off in the future and precious little was known about the functional anatomy of the frontal lobes? Favoring the shotgun over the rifle, the Portuguese physicians carved out six spheres of brain tissue from each frontal lobe. If they were dissatisfied with the results—if the patient was still disruptive, for instance—then Lima might go back and slice out even more brain tissue.

In 1936, Moniz and Lima published the results of their first twenty leucotomies. Before the surgery, nine patients had depression, seven had schizophrenia, two had anxiety disorders, and two were manic-depressive. Moniz claimed that seven patients improved significantly, another seven were somewhat improved, and the remaining six were unchanged. None, according to the authors, were worse off after the procedure.

When Moniz presented his results at a medical conference in Paris, Portugal's top psychiatrist, José de Matos Sobral Cid, denounced the new technique. Cid was director of psychiatry at Moniz's hospital and had viewed the leucotomized patients firsthand. He described them as "diminished" and exhibiting a "degradation of personality," and argued that their apparent improvement was actually shock, no different from what a soldier experienced after a severe head injury.

Moniz was undaunted. He also proposed a theory to explain why leucotomies worked, a theory firmly in the camp of biological psychiatry. He announced that mental illness resulted from "functional fixations" in the brain. These occurred when the brain could not stop performing the same activity over and over, and Moniz asserted that the leucotomy cured patients by eliminating their functional fixations. Cid decried Moniz's after-the-fact theory as "pure cerebral mythology."

Despite such criticisms, Moniz's treatment, the transcranial frontal leucotomy, was celebrated as a miracle cure, and the reason is understandable, if not quite forgivable. One of the most common problems for any asylum psychiatrist was how to manage disruptive patients. The asylum, after all, was designed to care for individuals who were too obstreperous to live in society on their own. But short of physically restraining them, how can you control a person who is persistently agitated, rowdy, and violent? For the alienists, the calming effects of Moniz's leucotomy seemed like the answer to their prayers. After a relatively simple surgery, endlessly troublesome patients could be rendered docile and obedient.

Leucotomies spread like wildfire through the asylums of both Europe and America (in the United States, they became popularly known as lobotomies). The adoption of Moniz's surgery transformed mental institutions in one way that was immediately apparent to the most casual visitor. For centuries, the standard asylum soundtrack consisted of incessant noise and commotion. Now, this boisterous din was replaced with a more agreeable hush. While most proponents of psychosurgery were aware of the dramatic changes in its subjects' personalities, they argued that Moniz's "cure" was at least more humane than locking patients in straitjackets or padded cells for weeks on end, and it was certainly more convenient for the hospital staff. Patients who had previously smacked the walls, hurled their food, and shouted at invisible specters now sat placidly, disturbing no one. Among the more notable people subjected to this dreadful treatment were Tennessee Williams's sister Rose and Rosemary Kennedy, the sister of President John F. Kennedy.

All too quickly, the American lobotomy evolved from a

method for subduing the most disruptive patients to a general therapy for managing all manner of mental illnesses. This trend followed the trajectory of so many other psychiatric movements—from Mesmerism to psychoanalysis to orgonomy— whose practitioners came to regard a narrowly prescribed method as a universal panacea. If the only tool you own is a hammer, the whole world looks like a nail.

On January 17, 1946, an American named Walter Freeman introduced a radical new method of psychosurgery. Freeman was an ambitious and highly trained neurologist who admired Moniz for his "sheer genius." He believed that mental illness resulted from overactive emotions that could be dampened by surgically lesioning the emotional centers of the brain. Freeman felt that many more patients could benefit from the procedure, if only it could be made more convenient and inexpensive: The Moniz method required a trained surgeon, an anesthesiologist, and a pricey hospital operating room. After experimenting with an ice pick and a grapefruit, Freeman ingeniously adapted Moniz's technique so that it could be performed in clinics, doctor's offices, or even the occasional hotel room.

On January 17, 1946, in his Washington, DC, office, Walter Freeman performed the first-ever "transorbital lobotomy," on a twenty-seven-year old woman named Sallie Ellen Ionesco. The procedure involved lifting the patient's upper eyelid and placing, under the eyelid and against the top of the eye socket, the point of a thin surgical instrument that closely resembled an ice pick. Next, a mallet was used to drive the point through the thin layer of bone at the back of the eye socket and into the brain. Then, like Moniz's coring procedure with a leucotome, the tip of the ice pick was rotated to create a lesion in the frontal lobe. Freeman performed ice pick lobotomies on no fewer than 2,500 patients in twenty-three states by the time of his death in 1972.

Transorbital lobotomies were still being performed when I entered medical school. My sole encounter with a lobotomized

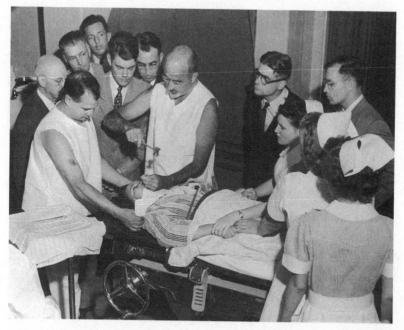

Walter Freeman performing a lobotomy. (© Bettmann/CORBIS)

patient was a rather cheerless affair. He was a thin, elderly man in St. Elizabeths Hospital in Washington, DC, who sat staring out at nothing in particular, as still as a granite statue. If you asked him a question, he responded in a quiet, robotic tone. If you made a request, he complied as dutifully as a zombie. Most disconcerting were his eyes, which appeared lifeless and blank. I was informed that at one time he had been unremittingly aggressive and unruly. Now, he was the "perfect" patient: obedient and low-maintenance in every way.

Astonishing though it may seem, Moniz received the Nobel Prize in 1949 "for his discovery of the therapeutic value of leucotomy in certain psychoses," marking the second Nobel Prize given for the treatment of mental illness. The fact that the Nobel committee was honoring malaria cures and lobotomies underscores the desperation for any form of psychiatric treatment.

Fortunately, contemporary psychiatry has long since discarded the dangerous and desperate methods of fever therapy, coma therapy, and transorbital lobotomies after the revolution in treatments beginning in the 1950s and '60s. But one form of therapy from the "snake pit" era has survived as the most common and effective somatic treatment in psychiatry today.

Electrified Brains

As the use of fever therapy and coma therapy spread through mental hospitals around the world, alienists observed another unexpected phenomenon: The symptoms of psychotic patients who also suffered from epilepsy seemed to improve after a seizure. Since fever improved the symptoms of patients with GPI, and insulin dampened the symptoms of psychosis, might seizures also be harnessed as a treatment?

In 1934, the Hungarian psychiatrist Ladislas J. Meduna began experimenting with different methods for inducing seizures in his patients. He tried camphor, a scented wax used as a food additive and embalming fluid, and then metrazol, a stimulant that causes seizures in high doses. Amazingly, Meduna discovered that psychotic symptoms really did diminish after a metrazol-induced seizure.

Meduna's novel seizure treatment quickly became known as *convulsive therapy*, and by 1937 the first international meeting on convulsive therapy was held in Switzerland. Within three years, metrazol convulsive therapy had joined insulin coma therapy as a standard treatment for severe mental illness in institutions all around the world.

There were problems with metrazol, however. First, before the convulsions actually started, the drug induced a feeling of impending doom in the patient, a morbid apprehension that was only heightened by the awareness that he was about to experience an uncontrollable seizure. This fearful anxiety must have been even worse for a psychotic patient already suffering from frightening delusions. Metrazol also provoked. thrashing convulsions so violent that they could become, quite literally, backbreaking. In 1939, an X-ray study at the New York State Psychiatric Institute found that 43 percent of patients who underwent metrazol convulsive therapy experienced fractures in their vertebrae.

Physicians began to look for a better way to induce seizures. In the mid-1930s, an Italian professor of neuropsychiatry, Ugo Cerletti, was experimentally inducing seizures in dogs by delivering electrical shocks directly to their heads. He wondered if electrical shocks might also induce seizures in humans, but his colleagues dissuaded him from attempting such experiments on people. Then one day while buying meat from the local butcher he learned that while slaughtering pigs, butchers often applied electrical shocks to their heads to put the animals into a kind of anesthetized coma before cutting their throats. Cerletti wondered: Would an electrical shock to a patient's head also produce anesthesia before provoking convulsions?

Before you decry Cerletti's project as wanton barbarism, it is worth reviewing the circumstances that led a trained doctor to consider running electricity through a person's brain—a notion, absent context, that sounds as terrifyingly absurd as the suggestion that dropping a pile of bricks on your toes will cure athlete's foot. First, there was still no effective treatment for severe mental illness besides insulin coma therapy and metrazol seizure therapy—dangerous, volatile, and highly invasive treatment. Second, for most patients, the only alternative to these extreme therapies was permanent institutionalization within a soul-crushing asylum. After watching shocked pigs become oblivious to the butcher's knife, Cerletti decided that shooting 100 volts of electricity through a person's skull was worth the obvious risks.

In 1938, Cerletti called upon his colleague Lucino Bini to build the first device explicitly designed to deliver therapeutic shocks to humans and, with Bini's collaboration, tried the device on their first patients. It worked just as Cerletti dreamed: The shock anesthetized each patient so that when he woke up he showed no memory of the seizure—and, as with metrazol, the patients showed marked improvement upon waking.

Beginning in the 1940s, Cerletti and Bini's technique, dubbed *electroconvulsive therapy,* or ECT, was adopted by almost every major psychiatric institution around the world. ECT was a welcome replacement for metrazol therapy because it was less expensive, less frightening to patients (no more feelings of impending doom), less dangerous (no more broken backs), more convenient (just flick the machine on and off)—and more effective. Depressed patients in particular often showed dramatic improvements in mood after just a few sessions, and while there were still some side effects to ECT, they were nothing compared to the daunting risks of coma therapy, malaria therapy, or lobotomies. It was truly a miracle treatment.

One of the side effects of ECT was retrograde amnesia, though many doctors considered this a perk rather than a drawback, since forgetting about the procedure spared patients any unpleasant memories of being electrocuted. Another side effect was due to the fact that early ECT procedures were usually administered in "unmodified form"—a euphemistic way of saying that the psychiatrists didn't use any kind of anesthesia or muscle relaxants—which resulted in full-scale convulsions that could produce bone fractures, though these were far less frequent and damaging than those resulting from metrazol-induced seizures. The introduction of suxamethonium, a synthetic alternative to curare, combined with a short-acting anesthetic, led to the widespread adoption of a much safer and milder "modified form" of ECT.

One of the earliest practitioners of ECT in the United

States was Lothar Kalinowsky, a German-born psychiatrist who immigrated to the United States in 1940. He settled in Manhattan, where he practiced psychiatry and neurology for more than forty years. I first met Kalinowsky as a resident in 1976 when he lectured and instructed the residents in ECT at St. Vincent's Hospital. A slender man with silver-gray hair and a heavy German accent, he was always immaculately attired, usually in a well-tailored three-piece suit, and carried himself with a dignified manner and professorial posture. I received excellent training in electroconvulsive therapy from the man who pioneered its use in American psychiatry.

To a young medical resident, the experience of delivering ECT can be quite disturbing. Since medical students are exposed to the same cultural stereotype of shock therapy as everyone else—that it is gruesome and barbaric—when you administer ECT for the very first time your conscience is pricked with the unsettling feeling that you are doing something wrong. A moral tension mounts inside you, and you must keep reminding yourself that extensive research and data support the therapeutic effects of ECT. But once you've seen the astonishingly restorative effects of ECT on a severely troubled patient, it all gets much easier. This is no lobotomy, producing vacant zombies. Patients are smiling and thanking you for the treatment. The experience is much like a medical student's first attempt at surgery: Cutting into a patient's abdomen and fishing around for an abscess or tumor can be gruesome and unnerving, but you must harm the patient a little in order to help him a lot—or even save his life.

Psychiatric treatment is not known for producing rapid results. Medical school lore holds that if you want to go into psychiatry you must be able to tolerate delayed gratification. Surgeons see the results of their treatment almost immediately after they stitch up an incision; for psychiatrists, waiting for drugs or psychotherapy to kick in is like watching ice melt. Not so with ECT. I've seen patients nearly comatose with depression joyfully bound off their cot within minutes of completing their ECT.

Whenever I think of ECT, one particular case comes to mind. Early in my career I treated the wife of a well-known New York restaurateur. Jean Claude was charismatic, cultured, and dedicated to his enormously successful French eatery. Still, not even his beloved restaurant came before his wife, Genevieve. She was a beautiful middle-aged woman who had once been a talented actress and still played the part of an ingénue. She also suffered from recurrent episodes of psychotic depression, a severe disorder that manifests with depressed mood, extreme agitation, and delusion-driven behavior. In the throes of an acute episode, she would become frantic, losing all control. Her usual impeccably mannered and charming demeanor would devolve into moaning and rocking. When her distress reached its crescendo, she would shudder and thrash her body in every direction, often shredding her clothes, and as if in counterpoint to her wild gyrations, Genevieve would break into loud baleful songs in her native French, sounding like a wounded Edith Piaf.

I first met Jean Claude when Genevieve was in the midst of one of her full-blown episodes. Other physicians had tried antidepressant and antipsychotic medications individually and in combination, with little effect. Rather than repeating the same medications, I suggested ECT. After the first session, Genevieve was calmer and screamed less, though she remained frightened and preoccupied. After several more treatments over the course of three weeks, she returned to her usual courteous self and thanked me, telling me this was the first time a psychiatrist had ever made her feel better. Jean Claude could not thank me enough and insisted that I dine at his restaurant whenever I wanted. I confess I took advantage of his offer and over the next couple of years I brought women I was dating to his chic gastronomic establishment whenever I wanted to make a good impression. One of these women became my wife.

Today, improved technologies enable ECT to be individually calibrated for each patient so that the absolute minimum amount of electrical current is used to induce a seizure. Moreover, the strategic placement of the electrodes at specific locations on the head can minimize side effects. Modern anesthetic agents combined with muscle relaxants and abundant oxygenation also render ECT an extremely safe procedure. ECT has been assiduously investigated over the past two decades, and the APA, NIH, and FDA all approve its use as a safe and effective treatment for patients with severe cases of depression, mania, or schizophrenia, and for patients who cannot take or do not respond to medication.

It strikes me as supremely ironic that the Nobel committee saw fit to award prizes for infecting patients with malaria parasites and for surgically destroying frontal lobes, two short-lived treatments that were neither safe nor effective, while passing over Cerletti and Bini despite the fact that their invention was the only early somatic treatment to become a therapeutic mainstay of psychiatry.

Despite the notable success of ECT, psychiatrists in the mid-twentieth century still yearned for a treatment that was cheap, noninvasive, and highly effective. But in 1950, such a therapy appeared to be nothing more than a pipe dream.

Chapter 6

Mother's Little Helper: Medicine at Last

Mother needs something today to calm her down
And though she's not really ill
There's a little yellow pill
She goes running for the shelter of a mother's little helper
— MICK JAGGER AND KEITH RICHARDS

It's better to be lucky than smart.
— HENRY SPENCER

Chloral Simmerings in My Spine

These days, it's difficult to imagine the practice of psychiatry without medication. You can hardly watch TV without seeing an ad for some mood-enhancing pill, usually featuring merry families frolicking on sandy beaches or joyous couples hiking through sun-dappled forests. Young people are far more likely to associate my profession with Prozac, Adderall, and Xanax than reclining on a couch week after week, divulging one's dreams and sexual fantasies. Schools, colleges, and nursing homes in every state openly endorse the liberal use of psychoactive drugs to mollify their more disruptive charges. What is less well known is that psychiatry's dramatic transformation from a profession of shrinks to a profession of pill-pushers came about through sheer serendipity.

When I was born, not a single therapeutically effective medication existed for any mental disorder. There were no antidepressants, no antipsychotics, no anti-anxiety drugs—at least, no sort of psychiatric drug that quelled your symptoms and enabled you to function effectively. The few existing treatments for the major categories of mental illness (mood disorders, schizophrenia, and anxiety disorders) were all invasive, risky, and burdened with appalling side effects, and these desperate measures were mostly used to control disruptive inmates in mental institutions. Similarly, the first psychiatric drugs were not intended to be curative or even therapeutic—they were blunt instruments for pacification. Their daunting side effects were only deemed acceptable because the alternatives—fever cures, coma therapy, induced convulsions—were even worse.

In the late nineteenth century, asylums used injections of *morphine* and other opiate-derived drugs to subdue recalcitrant inmates. While the patients may have ranked this among the most agreeable psychiatric treatments of the Victorian Era, the practice was discontinued once it became clear that opioids turned patients into hardcore addicts. The first behavior-altering drug commonly prescribed outside of asylums (*psychotropic drug,* in the argot of medicine) was *chloral,* a sleep-inducing non-opiate prescribed to relieve insomnia in anxious and depressed patients. Like morphine, chloral was not intended to treat a patient's most salient symptoms—namely, the fearfulness in anxiety disorders or the feelings of sadness in depression—it was intended to knock the patient out cold. Chloral was preferable to morphine because it was reliable in strength from dose to dose and could be given orally, but patients disliked its awful taste and the distinctive odor it imparted to their breath, known as "alky-breath."

Even though chloral was less addictive than morphine, it was still habit-forming. Women suffering from "nervous conditions" often self-administered the drug at home in order to avoid the embarrassment of institutionalization and frequently ended up as chloral addicts. The celebrated author Virginia

Woolf, who suffered from manic-depressive illness and was repeatedly institutionalized, frequently swallowed chloral in the 1920s. From her boudoir, she wrote to her lover Vita Sackville-West about its effects: "Goodnight now, I am so sleepy with chloral simmering in my spine that I can't write, nor yet stop writing—I feel like a moth, with heavy scarlet eyes and a soft cape of down—a moth about to settle in a sweet bush— would it were—ah, but that's improper."

Once its sleep-inducing properties became widely known, chloral quickly gained notoriety as perhaps the first drug employed to surreptitiously incapacitate a victim. Adding a few drops of chloral to someone's drink gave rise to the expression "slip him a mickey." (The term may have originally referred to a Chicago bartender, "Mickey" Finn, who added chloral to the drinks of customers he intended to rob.)

The simple act of putting a patient to sleep will inevitably reduce his symptoms. After all, when you lose consciousness, your anxieties, delusions, and manias subside, along with your nervous tics, ranting, and pacing. From this matter-of-fact observation, it was a short leap of imagination for psychiatrists to extrapolate the hypothesis that by prolonging their patients' sleep, they might diminish their symptoms during waking hours as well. Around the turn of the nineteenth century, Scottish psychiatrist Neil Macleod experimented on a variety of mental illnesses with a powerful sedative known as *sodium bromide.* He claimed that by rendering patients unconscious for an extended period of time, he could produce a complete remission of their mental disorders, a remission that sometimes lasted for days or even weeks. He called his treatment "deep sleep therapy"—an appealing moniker, for who doesn't feel rejuvenated after a restful slumber?

Unfortunately, there's quite a bit of difference between natural deep sleep and the sleep produced by a chemical strong enough to knock out an elephant. Deep sleep therapy can elicit a cauldron of scary side effects, including coma, cardiovascular collapse, and respiratory arrest; one of Macleod's own patients died during his experiments. It was also difficult to judge the right dose, and sometimes patients slept for a day or two longer than intended. Most problematic was the fact that bromide is a toxin that builds up in the liver, becoming more harmful with each use.

At first, bromide compounds spread rapidly through public asylums because they were cheaper and easier to manufacture than chloral, while producing more potent effects. The "bromide sleep cure" was briefly taken up by other physicians, too, before being abandoned as too dangerous.

Even though morphine, chloral, and bromide were all crude and addictive sedatives with harmful side effects, the notion that drug-induced sleep was therapeutic became firmly established by the start of World War II. (Except, of course, among the psychoanalysts, who dismissed sleeping pills out of hand, insisting they did nothing to resolve the unconscious conflicts that were the true mainspring of all mental illness.) Even so, no psychiatrist, psychoanalyst or otherwise, believed that there would ever be a drug that targeted the symptoms of mental illness or empowered a patient to lead a normal life — at least, not until 1950, the year the first *psychopharmaceutical* drug was born, a drug providing true therapeutic benefits for a troubled mind.

Despite the drug's momentous impact, I'd wager you've probably never heard of it: *meprobamate*. Originally marketed as Miltown, this synthetic medication alleviated anxiety and elicited a feeling of calm without putting patients to sleep. In the first peer-reviewed article describing meprobamate, the author characterized its effects as "tranquilizing," giving rise to the name of the first class of psychopharmaceuticals: *tranquilizers*.

Psychoanalysts denigrated meprobamate as just another chemical distraction that concealed mental illness rather than treating it, but the Freudians were the only ones to pooh-pooh it: meprobamate wasn't merely the world's first psychopharmaceutical, it was the world's first psychotropic blockbuster. By 1956, an astonishing 36 million prescriptions for the tranquilizer had been written; one out of every three prescriptions in the United States was for meprobamate. It was prescribed for everything from psychosis to addiction and came to be associated with overwrought housewives—giving rise to its popular sobriquet, "Mother's Little Helper," immortalized by the Rolling Stones.

Meprobamate was superseded in the 1960s by the introduction of Librium and Valium, a new generation of internationally popular tranquilizers. (The bestselling contemporary benzodiazepines are Xanax, for anxiety, and Ambien, for sleep.) All of these drugs trace their origins to Macleod's deep sleep therapy at the dawn of the twentieth century.

While meprobamate was unquestionably effective in reducing the symptoms of mild anxiety disorders, it was not a pharmaceutical game-changer like antibiotics for bacterial infections, insulin for diabetes, or vaccines for infectious diseases. It had no effect on the disturbing hallucinations, painful melancholy, or frenzied mania of patients locked away in public asylums, so it offered no hope for recovery for those unfortunate souls suffering from severe mental illness. Even after meprobamate become a psychiatric smash hit, the prospect of finding a simple pill that could ameliorate psychosis seemed as fanciful as schizophrenics' delusions and as remote as the asylums that imprisoned them.

Laborit's Drug

In 1949 a French surgeon named Henri Laborit was seeking a way to reduce surgical shock—the low blood pressure and rapid heart rate that often occurs after major surgery. According to one of the prevailing hypotheses at the time, surgical shock was due to the excessive reaction of a patient's autonomic nervous system to stress. (The autonomic nervous system is the unconscious circuitry that controls our breathing, heart rate, blood pressure, and other vital functions of the body.) Laborit believed that if he could find a compound that suppressed the autonomic nervous system, it would increase the safety of surgical procedures.

Working in a French military hospital in Tunisia—not exactly the epicenter of the medical world—Laborit experimented with a group of compounds called antihistamines. Today these drugs are commonly used to treat allergies and cold symptoms, but at the time scientists had just learned that antihistamines affect the autonomic system. Laborit noticed that when he gave a strong dose of one particular antihistamine, known as *chlorpromazine*, to his patients before surgery, their attitudes changed markedly: They became indifferent toward their imminent operation, an apathy that continued after the surgery was completed. Laborit wrote about this discovery, "I asked an army psychiatrist to watch me operate on some of my tense, anxious Mediterranean-type patients. Afterwards, he agreed with me that the patients were remarkably calm and relaxed."

Impressed by the notable psychological effects of the drug, Laborit wondered if chlorpromazine might be used to manage psychiatric disturbances. Pursuing his hunch, in 1951 Laborit administered a dose of chlorpromazine intravenously to a healthy psychiatrist at a French mental hospital who volunteered to serve as a human guinea pig in order to provide feedback about the drug's mental effects. At first the psychiatrist reported "no effects worthy of mention, save a certain sensation of indifference." But then, as he got up to go to the toilet, he fainted—the result of a drop in blood pressure, a side effect. After that, the director of the hospital's psychiatric service banned further experimentation with chlorpromazine.

Undeterred, Laborit attempted to persuade a group of psychiatrists at another hospital to test the drug on their psychotic patients. They were not particularly enthusiastic about his proposal, since the prevailing belief was that the disruptive symptoms of schizophrenia could only be reduced by strong sedatives, and chlorpromazine was not a sedative. But Laborit persevered and finally convinced a skeptical psychiatrist to try his drug on a schizophrenic patient.

On January 19, 1952, chlorpromazine was administered to Jacques L., a highly agitated twenty-four-year-old psychotic prone to violence. Following the drug's intravenous administration, Jacques rapidly settled down and became calm. After three steady weeks on chlorpromazine, Jacques carried out all his normal activities. He even played an entire game of bridge. He responded so well, in fact, that his flabbergasted physicians discharged him from the hospital. It was nothing short of miraculous: A drug had seemingly wiped away the psychotic symptoms of an unmanageable patient and enabled him to leave the hospital and return to the community.

What distinguished the effects of chlorpromazine so dramatically from sedatives and tranquilizers was its ability to decrease the intensity of psychotic symptoms — the hallucinations, delusions, and disorganized thinking — in the same way that aspirin reduces the pain of a headache or the temperature of a fever. A friend of mine who suffers from schizophrenia, the legal scholar Elyn Saks, writes in her memoir, *The Center Cannot Hold: My Journey Through Madness*, that antipsychotic drugs act more like a dimmer knob than an on/off switch. When her symptoms are at their worst, they cause her to hear sharp voices hurling painful insults at her or shouting orders she must obey; the meds gradually reduce her symptoms to a point where she still hears voices, but they are distant, faint, receding into the background and no longer distressing or compelling.

Chlorpromazine's use as an antipsychotic—the *first* antipsychotic—swept through the mental hospitals of Europe with the force of a tidal wave. In the psychoanalysis-obsessed United States, in contrast, reaction to the miracle med was muted. The Smith, Kline and French pharmaceutical company (a forerunner to GlaxoSmithKline) licensed chlorpromazine for distribution in the U.S., where it was endowed with the American trade name Thorazine (in Europe it was called Largactil), and launched a major marketing campaign to convince medical schools and psychiatry departments to test it on their patients. But American shrinks derided Laborit's drug as "psychiatric aspirin," waving it off as just another sedative, like chloral or the barbiturates—a distracting siren song that led gullible psychiatrists away from their true task of digging for neurotic seeds buried in the soil of the unconscious.

At first, Smith, Kline and French was baffled and frustrated by chlorpromazine's stony reception. They had in their possession a wonder drug proven to treat the symptoms of psychosis for the first time in human history, yet they couldn't convince anybody in America of its value. They finally stumbled upon a winning strategy: Rather than targeting psychiatrists with promises of a marvelous cure, they targeted state governments using a surprisingly modern argument. Referring to "health economics" and "cost-cutting," Smith, Kline and French argued that if state-funded mental institutions used chlorpromazine, they would be able to discharge patients instead of warehousing them forever. A few of these institutions—more concerned with the bottom line than with philosophical debates about the ultimate nature of mental illness—tried out Thorazine on their permanent patients. The results were breathtaking, just as French psychiatrists had previously demonstrated and Smith, Kline and French had promised. All but the most hopeless cases improved, and many long-institutionalized patients were sent home. After that, chlorpromazine took American psychiatry by storm. Every asylum and psychiatric hospital began to use Laborit's drug as the first line of treatment for psychotic patients in their care. Over the next fifteen years, Smith, Kline and French's revenues doubled three times. By 1964, more than ten thousand peer-reviewed articles had been published on chlorpromazine, and more than fifty million people around the world had taken the drug.

It is hard to overstate the epochal nature of Laborit's discovery. Like a bolt from the blue, here was a medication that could relieve the madness that disabled tens of millions of men and women—souls who had so very often been relegated to permanent institutionalization. Now they could return home and, incredibly, begin to live stable and even purposeful lives. They had a chance to work, to love, and—possibly—to have a family.

Just as the antibiotic streptomycin emptied sanitariums of tuberculosis patients and the polio vaccine rendered the iron lung obsolete, the widespread adoption of chlorpromazine marked the beginning of the end for the asylums. It also marked the end of the alienists. It is no coincidence that the asylum population began to decline from its peak in the United States in the same year Thorazine was released.

A century and a half after Philippe Pinel freed the inmates of the Parisian Hospice de la Salpêtrière from their physical chains, another French physician released patients from their mental confinement. Psychiatry, after a seemingly interminable struggle, could finally answer the question, "How can we treat severe mental illness?"

Compound G 22355

Envious of the mega-profits generated by chlorpromazine, other pharmaceutical companies searched for their own proprietary antipsychotic throughout the 1950s. They often teamed up with psychiatrists to aid in this search, and the Swiss pharmaceutical company Geigy, a corporate ancestor of Novartis, approached Roland Kuhn, the head doctor at a psychiatric hospital in the Swiss town of Münsterlingen, on the banks of Lake Constance. Kuhn, thirty-eight, was a tall and cultivated psychiatrist who combined an exceptional grasp of the humanities with a background in biochemistry. Geigy offered to provide Kuhn with experimental compounds if he would test them on his patients. Kuhn readily agreed.

In late 1955, Geigy's head of pharmacology met Kuhn at a hotel in Zurich where he showed him a chart scribbled with the hand-drawn chemical structures of forty different compounds available for testing. "Pick one," the pharmacologist instructed. Kuhn carefully surveyed the forest of molecules, then pointed to the one that most closely resembled chlorpromazine, a molecule labeled "Compound G 22355."

Kuhn dosed a few dozen psychotic patients with G 22355, but the drug failed to produce the same dramatic reduction of symptoms as chlorpromazine. Of course, as any pharmacological researcher knows, failure is the usual fate for any experimental compound—most commercial drugs are only discovered after tens of thousands or even hundreds of thousands of chemical candidates are tested and rejected. The most sensible next step would have been for Kuhn to point to a new compound on Geigy's chart and try again. Instead, Kuhn made a very peculiar decision, one that would affect millions of lives.

The first antipsychotic was not discovered because of any orderly research plan contrived by Big Pharma; it was discovered purely by accident after a solitary physician followed his intuition about an experimental drug for surgical shock. And now a lone psychiatrist decided to ignore the task that he had been assigned—finding a chlorpromazine knockoff—and instead pursued his own private hunch about a disorder he cared about more than schizophrenia: depression.

Even in the earliest days of psychiatry, schizophrenia and depression were almost always considered distinct conditions; madness and melancholia. After all, the worst symptoms of psychosis were cognitive, while the worst symptoms of depression were emotional. When Geigy engaged Kuhn, there was no reason to believe that a class of drugs that dampened the hallucinations of psychotic patients would also elevate the mood of depressed patients. But Kuhn held his own staunch ideas about the nature of depression.

Kuhn rejected the standard psychoanalytic explanation that depressed individuals were suffering from buried anger toward their parents, so he didn't believe depression should be treated with psychotherapy. On the contrary: he shared the assumption of biological psychiatrists that depression resulted from some unidentifiable neural dysfunction. Nevertheless, Kuhn disliked the prevailing "biological" treatment for depression, sleep therapy; he felt it failed to target the symptoms of depression, instead relying on crude chemical force to bludgeon the patient's entire consciousness. Kuhn wrote to a colleague, "How often I thought we should improve the opium treatment. But how?"

Without telling Geigy, Kuhn administered G 22355 to three patients suffering from severe depression. After a few days, the patients showed no signs of improvement. This stood in sharp contrast to sedatives like morphine or chloral or even chlorpromazine itself, which produced often drastic effects within hours or even minutes of administration. For reasons known only to Kuhn, he continued administering G 22355 to his patients anyway. On the morning of the sixth day of treatment, January 18, 1956, a patient named Paula woke up feeling quite changed.

The nurses reported that Paula exhibited more energy and was uncharacteristically talkative and sociable. When Kuhn examined her, her melancholy was remarkably improved, and for the first time she expressed optimism for her future. This was just as astonishing as Laborit's first patient, Jacques L., playing a full game of bridge. Some days after Paula, the other two patients also began to manifest thrilling signs of recovery. Kuhn enthusiastically wrote to Geigy about his unauthorized experiment, "The patients feel less tired, the sensation of weight decreases, the inhibitions become less pronounced, and the mood improves."

Incredibly, Geigy expressed no interest in Kuhn's discovery. The company was fixated on finding an antipsychotic to compete with chlorpromazine, not exploring some radical and unknown treatment for melancholia. Ignoring Kuhn completely, Geigy hurriedly sent G 22355 to other psychiatrists and ordered them to test the compound exclusively on schizophrenics, never mentioning its potential effects on depression. Geigy executives snubbed Kuhn again the next year, when he attended a psychopharmacology conference in Rome and repeated his request to pursue G 22355 as a depression-fighting drug. Kuhn's lonesome discovery seemed destined for the scrap heap of medical history.

He tried to interest other academics, but they, too, collectively shrugged their shoulders. When Kuhn presented a paper on G 22355 at a scientific meeting in Berlin, only a dozen people showed up. After he finished his talk—in which he described the world's first effective pharmacological treatment for depression—none of the attendees asked a single question.

One person in the audience was Frank Ayd, an American psychiatrist and devout Catholic, who told me years later, "Kuhn's words, like those of Jesus, were not appreciated by those in positions of authority. I don't know if anybody in that room appreciated we were hearing the announcement of a drug that would revolutionize the treatment of mood disorders."

But as with Laborit's drug, fate—or blind luck—intervened once again. An influential Geigy stockholder and business partner named Robert Boehringer knew of Kuhn's expertise in mood disorders and asked if he could suggest anything for his wife, who was suffering from depression. Without hesitation, Kuhn recommended G 22355—and made sure to point out that the stockholder's company was refusing to develop the drug. After taking the experimental compound for a week, Mrs. Boehringer's depression lifted. Delighted, Boehringer began lobbying Geigy executives to develop the drug as an antidepressant. Under pressure from such an influential partner (Boehringer also owned his own pharmaceutical enterprise), Geigy changed course and began formal human trials of G 22355 on depressed patients and finally bestowed the compound with its own name: *imipramine.*

In 1958, Geigy released imipramine to the public. It was the first of a new class of drugs known as tricyclic antidepressants—so named because the compounds' molecular structure is composed of three joined molecular rings. (When a drug is named after its chemical structure rather than its physiological mechanism, it's a sure sign that nobody knows how it works. Another class of antidepressants are known as selective serotonin reuptake inhibitors, or SSRIs; needless to say, scientists have since learned they produce their effects by inhibiting neurons' reuptake of the neurotransmitter serotonin.) Unlike chlorpromazine, imipramine was an instant global success, equally embraced by psychiatrists in Europe and America.

Other pharmaceutical companies soon released a flood of tri-cyclic antidepressants, all knock-offs of imipramine.

It's not possible to overstate the prodigious impact of chlor-promazine and imipramine on the practice of psychiatry. Less than a decade after the release of Thorazine in the United States, the entire profession was utterly transmogrified. Two of its three flagship illnesses, schizophrenia and depression, were reclassified from "wholly untreatable" to "largely manageable." Only manic-depressive illness, the final mental scourge of humanity, remained bereft of treatment and hope.

Serendipity Down Under

As these accidental discoveries of miracle medications were occurring in Europe, an unknown doctor in an obscure cor-ner of the medical world was quietly pursuing his own profes-sional hobbyhorse: a cure for mania. John Cade was initially trained as a psychiatrist, but during World War II he served as a surgeon in the Australian Army. In 1942, he was captured by the Japanese during their conquest of Singapore and locked up at Changi Prison, where he observed many of his fellow prisoners of war exhibiting the unhinged behavior that so often accompanied combat trauma. They trembled, they shrieked, they babbled mindlessly. Struck by what he perceived as the similarity between these war-induced symptoms and those produced by mania, Cade hypothesized that the prison-ers' quasi-manic behavior might be caused by a stress-induced toxin produced by the body. Perhaps such medical specula-tions helped him endure the sweltering nights in his dank, cramped cell.

Cade was eventually released, and after the war he pursued his toxin theory of mania at the Bundoora Repatriation Mental

Hospital in Melbourne. His experiments were straightforward, if somewhat crude: He injected urine from manic patients into the abdomen of guinea pigs. Uric acid, found in urine, is a naturally occurring metabolite in humans. Excessive uric acid causes gout, and Cade guessed that uric acid might also cause mania if it accumulated in the brain. After the guinea pigs received a gut-full of human urine, Cade recorded that they exhibited "increased and erratic activity." He interpreted these manic-like behaviors as confirmation of his toxin theory, though an alternative interpretation might be that any creature will exhibit erratic activity after getting a syringe of foreign urine in its belly.

The next step, Cade reasoned, was to find a compound that would neutralize uric acid, the putative mania-producing toxin. Since uric acid is not soluble in water (this is why it accumulates in gout victims), he decided to add a chemical to the manic-derived urine that would dissolve the uric acid and help the guinea pigs (and, presumably, manic patients) excrete it more easily, thereby reducing the guinea pigs' mania.

Now, let's pause just a moment to put Cade's experiment into perspective. Henri Laborit, recall, was pursuing a (largely incorrect) theory of surgical shock when he stumbled upon the first antipsychotic drug entirely by accident. Roland Kuhn, for no logical reason, decided to find out if a psychosis-fighting compound might be better suited for lifting the spirits of the despondent, leading to the first antidepressant. From these examples it is clear that the process that led to such momentous discoveries was not a rational one, but rather, more guided by intuition and serendipity. And now, since metabolic toxins have absolutely nothing to do with mania, John Cade was pursuing the totally spurious hypothesis that mania could be eliminated by finding the right solvent to dissolve uric acid.

The solvent Cade selected was lithium carbonate, a compound known to dissolve uric acid. Cade first injected his guinea pigs with "manic urine," then injected them with lithium carbonate. To his delight, the previously "manic" guinea pigs soon became calm. Cade took this as further confirmation of his toxin theory—after all, weren't the guinea pigs quieting down because they were successfully excreting uric acid? Unfortunately for Cade, when he tested other uric acid solvents on the animals, they failed to produce any calming effects. Gradually, he realized that the guinea pigs' placated behavior was not because uric acid was getting dissolved—there was something special about the lithium itself.

To his credit as a scientist, Cade abandoned his toxin theory of mania, which his data simply didn't support. Instead, he threw himself wholeheartedly behind the development of lithium carbonate as a treatment for mental illness, without having any clue why it pacified hyperactive animals. In 1949, Cade conducted a small-scale trial of lithium on patients diagnosed with mania, psychosis, and melancholia. The effect on the frenzied behavior of the manic patients was nothing short of extraordinary. The calming effect was so robust that Cade came up with a new hypothesis: mania was caused by a physiological deficiency of lithium.

While Cade's second theory turned out to be as short-lived as his first, his treatment was not. Lithium proved to be a godsend, and today lithium is used around the world as a first-line drug to treat bipolar disorder. Left untreated—and before the discovery of lithium, bipolar disorder always went untreated— the illness is highly destructive to the brain and can sometimes be fatal, as illustrated by the untimely death of Philippe Pinel's friend. Another casualty of bipolar disorder was Philip Graham, the celebrated publisher of the *Washington Post*. On August 3, 1963, while on a brief leave from the Chestnut Lodge psychiatric hospital, where he was receiving psychoanalytic treatment for his manic-depressive illness, he went to his country home and killed himself with one of his hunting rifles. His widow, Katherine Graham, never forgave the psychiatric profession for failing him. Sadly, lithium was already available at the time of his death, though it was not approved for use in the U.S. until 1970.

When given in the proper dosage, lithium levels out the wild mood swings of bipolar disorder, permitting those suffering from the illness to live normal lives. To this day, lithium remains the most effective mood stabilizer (the name given to the class of medication for treating bipolar disorder), though alternative mood stabilizing drugs are now available.

By 1960—after a century and a half of groping in the darkness—psychiatry possessed reliable treatments for all three types of severe mental illness. What made chlorpromazine, imipramine, and lithium so different from the sedatives and tranquilizers that came before was that they directly targeted psychiatric symptoms in a kind of lock-and-key relationship. Sedatives and tranquilizers produced the same broad mental changes in everyone, whether or not a person suffered from a mental disorder, whereas antipsychotics, antidepressants, and mood stabilizers reduced the symptoms of illness without producing much of an effect on healthy people. Even better, the new drugs were not addictive and did not produce euphoria, like barbiturates or opiates. This meant the drugs were not particularly appealing to the worried well and did not become habit-forming in those suffering from mental illness.

Unfortunately, the fact that these new classes of drugs were not habit-forming meant that many patients did not feel compelled to continue taking them once their symptoms subsided, especially since chlorpromazine, imipramine, and lithium each had various unpleasant side effects, particularly if the doses were not carefully regulated. But for most patients (and their families), the side effects of psychopharmaceuticals were far outweighed by the near-miraculous relief from chronic, distressing symptoms.

I have experienced firsthand the unique effects of each class of psychopharmaceuticals. During my pharmacology class in medical school, my instructor assigned us to imbibe a series of medications during the semester, one dose each week. Every Friday we were given a small cup of liquid to swallow. Our assignment was to describe the effects we experienced over the following hour and then guess which drug it was. While we knew the possible choices—which included alcohol, amphetamine, the sedative Seconal, Valium, Thorazine, the antidepressant Tofranil, and a placebo—the identity of each drug was not revealed until we had completed the entire series. The results shocked me. I had guessed wrong on every single drug except for Thorazine; the antipsychotic had made my mind feel fatigued and dull, thinking demanded painful effort, and I felt indifferent to everything around me. Later, as a resident, I sampled lithium but didn't feel much of anything other than increased thirst and the paradoxical need to urinate.

The mind-boggling effectiveness of psychiatric drugs began to transform the fundamental nature of psychiatry—and elevate its professional status. The black sheep of medicine could rejoin the flock because it finally *had* medicine. President Kennedy, in his address to Congress in 1963, acknowledged the changing landscape of mental health: "The new drugs acquired and developed in recent years make it possible for most of the mentally ill to be successfully and quickly treated in their own communities and returned to a useful place in society. Such breakthroughs have rendered obsolete a prolonged or permanent confinement in huge, unhappy mental hospitals."

Needless to say, the transformation of psychiatry also transformed the psychiatrist.

The Pioneers of Psychopharmacology

At various moments during my undergraduate years at Miami University in Oxford, Ohio, I imagined myself as a surgeon, obstetrician, cardiologist, radiologist, neurologist, and, on occasion, as a psychiatrist. The writings of Sigmund Freud first introduced me to the medicine of the mind and the possibility of fathoming the most beguiling organ of the human body through thoughtful analysis. But a very different sort of encounter introduced me to the possibility of understanding the brain through biology, chemistry, and neural circuitry. While working on this book, I discovered that Bob Spitzer and I shared a common experience in our professional development—a youthful experiment with LSD.

Though taking mind-expanding drugs was something of a rite of passage for those coming of age in the '60s, I suspect that my own approach to dropping acid was rather atypical. In 1968, my junior year—the same year the Beatles released their psychedelic movie *Yellow Submarine* and a year before the Woodstock Festival in Bethel, New York—I decided to try psychedelic drugs. I didn't rush out to join the latest hippie "happening." Cautious by nature, I systematically considered the recreational drugs that were in popular use—marijuana, uppers, downers, hallucinogens—and weighed the pros and cons of each, the way most people might approach buying a new car. I decided that my (perhaps overambitious) goal was to expand my understanding of the world and illuminate the mystery that was myself. After reading several exciting counter-cultural books detailing the wild mind-expanding journeys evoked by hallucinogens, such as *The Varieties of Religious Experience, The Doors of Perception,* and *The Teachings of Don Juan,* I thought I had finally found the drug I was looking for—the sultan of psychedelics, lysergic acid diethylamide.

I decided to trip with my girlfriend Nancy and, characteristically, I fastidiously planned out every detail of the big event in advance. The LSD came in squares of absorbent paper, called blotter acid, and Nancy and I each swallowed two small squares (about 100 micrograms), then headed out onto campus on a warm spring afternoon. Within fifteen minutes, I felt a tingling sensation throughout my body, beginning in my abdomen and then welling up throughout my body. Soon, my visual, auditory, and tactile perceptions began to fluctuate and intensify. The grass and trees appeared brighter, the green almost spectacular in its vividness. My hands became objects of wonder, radiating kaleidoscopic patterns that oscillated in and out of focus. The ambient noise of the field we were crossing twisted through bewitching arpeggios of sound.

Eventually, as part of my planned itinerary, we arrived at a church near the campus and sat together in a pew. I marveled at the dazzling stained glass and the staggering beauty of the altar. Until then, the effects of the LSD had been mostly perceptual. Now a new experience emerged that was far more intense and mind-bending—in fact, I often recall this portion of my trip when I work with psychotic patients. As I gazed upon the religious accouterments of the church, I was filled with an overwhelming spiritual awareness, as if God was communicating His secret and divine meaning to me. A cascade of insights tumbled through my consciousness, seeming to touch my soul and thrilling me with their profundity. And then in the midst of this revelatory reverie, a disembodied voice whispered, "And no one will ever know," which seemed to signify to me that this was where the *real truths* lie, in these secret interstices of consciousness which most human beings never accessed—or if they did, they were unable to retain these precious encounters in their memory. I looked over at Nancy, assuming that she was immersed in the same transcendent, exalting experience as I was. "We must start coming to services here to maintain this spiritual connection!" I exclaimed. She looked at me querulously and barked, "But you're Jewish!"

We later realized that our individual experiences were entirely separate and often absurdly different. As my mind soared through metaphysical realms of empyrean knowledge, she spent most of her trip reflecting on her relationship with her father, an Episcopalian WASP whose ancestors came over on the *Mayflower,* ruminating fearfully on what he would say about her having a Jewish boyfriend.

But the most deflating moment came when I pulled out my written notes. During the trip, I had jotted down descriptions of my revelations, expecting to revisit these profound pearls of cosmic wisdom once the drug wore off. Now, as I scanned my chaotic scribbles, I found them either boringly mundane — "love is the essence" — or ludicrously nonsensical — "leaves are green clouds." Later, whenever I encountered Szasz or Laing or any other antipsychiatrist talking about the "journey of the schizophrenic," I recalled my private log of Great Thoughts. Just because a person *believes* he is having a cosmic encounter — whether because of drugs or mental illness — it doesn't mean he is.

My trip did produce one lasting insight, though — one that I remain grateful for to this day. Though my LSD-fueled reverie dissipated with the light of the morning, I marveled at the fact that such an incredibly minute amount of a chemical — 50 to 100 micrograms, a fraction of a grain of salt — could so profoundly affect my perceptions and emotions. It struck me that if LSD could so dramatically alter my cognition, the chemistry of the brain must be susceptible to pharmacologic manipulation in other ways, including ways that could be therapeutic. During an era when Freud still held dominion over American psychiatry, my psychedelic experiment opened me up to an alternative way of thinking about mental pathologies beyond psychodynamics—as something concrete and biochemical in the cellular coils of the brain.

Before chlorpromazine, imipramine, and lithium, severe mental illness was almost always a life sentence of misery and a source of great shame to the families of the afflicted. Making matters worse, the prevailing psychiatric theories blamed the parents for the way they raised their child, or the patients themselves for their "resistance to treatment." But the success of the psychopharmaceuticals challenged head-on the fundamental tenets of psychoanalysis. If depression was due to parental anger turned inward, if psychosis was due to demanding and confusing mothers, if mania was due to unresolved infantile grandiosity, then how could gulping down a small tablet make these symptoms fade away?

Psychiatric medication not only challenged everything psychoanalysts had ever been taught about mental illness—it threatened their very livelihood. Those psychoanalysts who did deign to prescribe the new drugs considered them to be a treatment of last resort, to be used only when psychotherapy had been tried and had failed. But along with many other psychiatrists from my generation—many of whom also experimented with psychedelic drugs—I became receptive to the unexpected new role of psychiatrists as *psychopharmacologists*, as empathic prescribers of medication.

The very first generation of psychopharmacologists had all been indoctrinated into the psychoanalytic tradition during their training but often harbored doubts about Freudian dogma. Not surprisingly, it was the youngest psychiatrists who most readily embraced the new psychiatric drugs. Starting in psychiatry departments in the 1960s, the pressure to use the new medications often came from residents who were still in training. Gradually, medications began to permeate clinical psychiatry, and practitioners who buoyantly advocated drug therapy became increasingly common.

The growing contingent of psychopharmacologists increased the number of biological psychiatrists to its largest since the heyday of Wilhelm Griesinger. To their medical colleagues in other specialties, the psychopharmacologists were a breath of fresh air; finally, there were medically minded psychiatrists to whom they could relate and confidently refer mental patients. But from the point of view of their psychoanalytic colleagues, these maverick psychopharmacologists were regarded as heretics and worse—the pitiable products of failed analyses, individuals who could not overcome their own conflicts, conflicts that made them defy Freud's masterful teachings and neurotically cling to the delusion that chemicals could cure patients.

Brash and outspoken, the psychopharmacologists didn't just voice a new and radical philosophy about mental illness; they behaved in forbidden ways. They refused to affect the deliberate manner of a proper analyst, who spoke in stilted and omniscient tones or quietly listened in a detached manner. Instead, they engaged their patients with lively and probative back-and-forth discussions and strove to be empathetic and even reassuring. Sometimes they saw patients for 30, 20, or even 15 minutes rather than the requisite 45- or 50-minute hour. Occasionally, in order to take someone's pulse or blood pressure, examine side effects, or just greet a patient with a handshake, they even committed the cardinal sin of touching their patients. These early heretics/pioneers included Jonathan Cole of Harvard, Frank Ayd of the University of Maryland, Sam Gershon of New York University, Donald Klein of Columbia, and—the most notorious apostate of them all— Nathan Kline.

Perhaps better than any other, the story of Kline's career illustrates the greatest triumphs of the first generation of psychopharmacologists—as well as their most egregious shortcomings. When Nathan Kline graduated from the NYU School of Medicine in 1943, psychiatry was a scientific wasteland parched by psychoanalytic theory. But Kline was too intellectually restless to engage in what he felt was a scientific charade, and early in his career he began searching for pharmaceutical treatments. At first, the only compounds available to a would-be psychopharmacologist were the various sedatives and tranquilizers, which he dutifully investigated. Frustrated by the lack of effective drugs, he expanded his search to other spheres of medicine. Intrigued by the use of the snakeroot plant (Rauvolfia serpentina) as a tranquilizer in India (Gandhi famously used it), he used a snakeroot extract called reserpine experimentally on schizophrenics in the early 1950s. Although his initial results were promising, they were abruptly eclipsed by the emergence of chlorpromazine.

Kline began investigating other novel psychoactive compounds. Eventually, in 1959, he published a groundbreaking series of studies of iproniazid, a drug used to treat tuberculosis, demonstrating its effectiveness as an antidepressant. Kline's studies established an entirely new class of antidepressants with a pharmacology distinct from imipramine called monoamine oxidase inhibitors (this time, scientists understood how the drug worked in the brain). This discovery launched Kline into the scientific stratosphere. His research accorded him the unique distinction of being the only scientist to ever win the prestigious Lasker Award twice.

As a flood of new psychiatric drugs began to be approved by the FDA in the late '50s and '60s, Kline eagerly tried out each one in his clinical practice in New York. Whereas most Manhattan psychiatrists of the era focused on endless sessions of Freudian talk therapy, Kline aggressively prescribed the very latest drugs, often in creative combinations, and dramatically reduced the length, number, and frequency of talk therapy sessions.

In 1960, *Life* magazine called Kline "a pioneer of the new drug therapies for mental illness." He was celebrated through-out medicine and elected to the most elite scientific societies. Perhaps more than any other single person, Nathan Kline was also responsible for the deinstitutionalization of patients from mental hospitals in New York State: Buoyed by the dra-matic results of his ongoing psychopharmacologic research, Kline supplied Governor Nelson Rockefeller with a vision of medication-driven community mental health care, an effort that dovetailed with President Kennedy's introduction of the Community Mental Health Act in 1963. Kline was sought out by celebrities and politicians for treatment and frequently lauded in the press. His meteoric rise demonstrated the transformative effects that drugs were having on psychiatry and mental health care—but it would also reveal the hazards that accompanied the rapid pharmaceuticalization of psychiatry.

Nathan Kline was at the height of his career when I first met him in 1977 at a psychopharmacology meeting sponsored by the National Institute of Mental Health in Florida. I was in my second year of residency training in psychiatry and had been dispatched to the Sonesta Hotel on Key Biscayne by my mentor to present the results of our investigation of a new antipsychotic drug.

The roughly three hundred attendees were a mix of aca-demic researchers and National Institute of Health scientists, along with representatives from pharmaceutical companies. On the evening of the first day's sessions, a cocktail reception was held on the terrace adjacent to the pool overlooking the beach. I approached the crowd and was struck by a memorable sight. On one side of the terrace was a rowdy group of conference-goers gabbling away in shorts, bathing suits, and T-shirts. On the other side, reclining on a chaise longue over-looking the ocean, was Nathan Kline, looking regal in an immaculate white tropical leisure suit, and surrounded by a coterie of attendants. He held a tropical drink in one hand as he directed his minions with the other, like a monarch granting an audience to his subjects.

Shortly before the conference I had read a report in the *Archives of General Psychiatry* about Kline's research with a new compound called beta-endorphin, which he had administered to schizophrenia patients with dramatic results. This was an astonishing finding, as the only known antipsychotics were all chemical variants of chlorpromazine, whereas beta-endorphin was a naturally occurring peptide that was produced by the body, a completely different kind of compound. After discovering an entirely new class of antidepressants (the MAO-inhibitors), it appeared that Kline had now discovered an entirely new class of antipsychotics.

I nervously walked over and introduced myself. I asked him several questions about his study, as much to impress him with my knowledge as to deepen my understanding of his. At first he greeted me warily, but after realizing that I was a genuine admirer he warmed up and responded enthusiastically. He concluded by thanking me magisterially for my questions.

Only later did I learn that despite his fame, Kline had become something of a pariah in scientific circles. In modern parlance, he had "jumped the shark." It should have been apparent to me at the Florida conference that his pompous behavior would be alienating to his colleagues, but as a young resident I was naïve and starstruck. I would soon learn first-hand his sins against the medical codes of conduct.

As I continued my residency at St. Vincent's Hospital in Manhattan, I began to encounter what many psychiatrists in New York dubbed the "Kline experience." Patients of Dr. Kline began to drift into the emergency room and the outpatient clinic, and as new admissions to the psychiatric inpatient unit. All were victims of Kline's risky and sometimes heedless

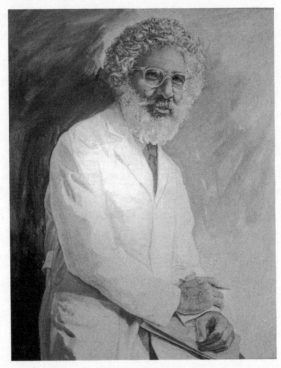

Nathan Kline (1916–83), a flamboyant pioneer of psychopharmacol-
ogy. (Portrait of Dr. Kline by David Laska, courtesy of Dr. Eugene
Laska and the Nathan S. Kline Institute for Psychiatric Research,
Orangeburg, NY; photograph courtesy of Koon-Sea Hui, MPhil, PhD)

practice. They suffered from severe adverse reactions caused
by elaborate cocktails of psychotropic medications—or from
the effects of their abrupt withdrawal. Whereas most psychiatrists treated depression, bipolar disorder, schizophrenia, or
anxiety disorders by prescribing one or two medications, possibly three on a rare occasion, Dr. Kline frequently prescribed
extravagant combinations of five or more medications in their
most potent forms, often at high doses. It got to the point
where I was able to guess whether a patient was one of Kline's
simply by glancing at the list of medications on his chart. No

one else had the confidence—or recklessness—to prescribe such witches' brews of mind-altering cocktails.

In the end, it was not the death of a patient or a massive malpractice suit that prompted Kline's downfall, though that was surely a possibility. It was the very study that had inspired me to timidly seek an audience with him in Florida. Kline had failed to submit the protocol for his study to an Institutional Review Board for approval, an ethical and legal requirement when conducting medical research on human subjects. Not only that, he hadn't bothered to get the proper informed consent from the patients to whom he was administering experimental psychoactive compounds. Apparently, in his eagerness to achieve another stunning scientific success (and perhaps win a Nobel), he had rushed to be the very first researcher to publish on a potential new class of psychopharmaceutical.

The FDA investigated Kline, and in 1982 he was compelled to sign a federal consent decree swearing to never conduct research on drugs again. Psychoactive drugs had launched Kline's career—and they ended it in ignominy. A year later, he died on an operating table from complications arising from an aortic aneurysm.

Despite Kline's excesses, the advent of psychopharmacology had irrevocably changed the field of psychiatry for the better. Those suffering from severe mental illness now could hope for relief and genuine recovery. But it also created tensions in a field struggling to redefine itself. This quandary was not lost on the media, which laid bare the emerging ideological fault lines. In 1955, in the wake of chlorpromazine's redesign of the mental health landscape, *Time* magazine reported, "The ivory-tower critics (mainly psychoanalysts) argue that the red-brick pragmatists—state hospitals—are not getting to the patients' 'underlying psychopathology' and so there can be no cure. These doctors want to know whether he withdrew from the world because of unconscious conflict over incestuous urges or stealing from his brother's piggy bank at the age of five. In the world of red-bricks, this is like arguing about the number of angels on the point of a pin."

But before the psychopharmacologists could permanently tip the balance away from the ivory-tower psychoanalysts, one final revolution was still necessary.

Part III

Psychiatry Reborn

If there is one central intellectual reality at the end of the twentieth century, it is that the biological approach to psychiatry — treating mental illness as a genetically influenced disorder of brain chemistry — has been a smashing success. Freud's ideas, which dominated the history of psychiatry for much of the past century, are now vanishing like the last snows of winter.

— EDWARD SHORTER

Chapter 7

Out of the Wilderness: The Brain Revolution

Here is this three-pound mass of jelly you can hold in the palm of your hand, and it can contemplate the vastness of interstellar space. It can contemplate the meaning of infinity and it can contemplate itself contemplating on the meaning of infinity.

— VILAYANUR RAMACHANDRAN

Every pusillanimous creature that crawls on the earth or slinks through slimy seas has a brain!

— THE WIZARD OF OZ

If I Only Had a Brain

In *The Wizard of Oz*, the Scarecrow yearns for a brain. To his surprise, the Wizard informs him that he already possesses one—he just doesn't know it. For most of the twentieth century, the same might have been said about psychiatry—it was brainless. Though ostensibly a medical specialty devoted to abnormalities of thought and emotion, psychiatry did not turn its attention to the *organ* of thought and emotion until the 1980s.

Psychiatrists were not alone in ignoring the brain—the level of interest in the pinkish stuffing inside our heads has long been woefully disproportionate to its importance, especially when compared to its main rival for anatomical preeminence: the heart. When we marry or fall in love, we give our *heart* to another, but never our brain. When someone leaves us we feel *heartbroken*, not *brainbroken*. Generous people are said to have *big hearts* or be *good-hearted* or have *hearts of gold* rather than *brains of gold*. Even the Bible invests the heart with psychic properties: "And you shall love the Lord your God with all your heart."

But the heart is nothing more than a glorified pump. Its sole function is to contract and expand, over and over, two billion times over the average lifespan, pushing blood through the body. In contrast, the human brain is an unfathomable supercomputer that exceeds every other organ in complexity by many orders of magnitude. Starting as an unimaginably tiny neural tube forming three weeks after conception, the brain grows at an astonishingly rapid pace to become a three-pound corrugated doughlike lump—comprising a hundred billion neurons communicating through thirty trillion connections— that somehow regulates our heart rate, body temperature, and appetite while simultaneously driving us to sing melodies, sculpt statues, code software...and pen lengthy treatises about itself. Comparing the heart to the brain is like comparing a child's dollhouse to New York City.

One thing that has always confounded any researcher wishing to scrutinize the brain is the fact that this arcane supermachine is encased within an impenetrable vessel: the skull. Until very recently, the only way to actually *examine* a thinking, feeling brain was through extremely invasive procedures or by carving up a lifeless brain at autopsy. It's not very surprising that the first science-tinged theory of the brain was founded on a rather ingenious (if completely misguided) method of circumventing the need to directly access the brain: *phrenology.*

Developed by the German physician Franz Joseph Gall in 1809, phrenology took as its starting point the assumption that different parts of the brain controlled specific functions. One region controlled hunger, another controlled lust, another anger. As neuroscientists would later confirm, this assumption turned out to be largely correct: specific mental functions are indeed localized in specific brain regions. Gall's next two hypotheses were not so lucky, though. He believed that if a person exhibited disproportionate activity issuing from a particular mental function—excessive lust, for instance—then (1) the part of his brain that governed lust would be enlarged, and (2) the skull above this enlarged part of his brain would also be enlarged. Thus, Gall claimed it was possible to discern a person's true psychological constitution by measuring the relative size of the various bumps and indentations on his head. You might say that phrenology was the world's first crude attempt at brain mapping.

Gall diligently appraised the skull geometries of prisoners, hospital patients, and asylum lunatics, and reported many sensational "findings." The heads of the stark raving mad featured a depression toward the back of their skull, which Gall interpreted as indicating a diminishment of their faculty of self-control. Young thieves possessed bumps just above their ears. All of these purported correlations between skull geometries and behavior turned out to be completely groundless. We now know there is no connection between a person's personality and the shape of his head.

Unable to provide any useful predictions about human behavior, phrenology had completely fallen out of favor by the middle of the nineteenth century, about the same time that Wilhelm Griesinger declared that mental illnesses were "illnesses of the nerves and brain."

A century later, in the late 1940s and '50s, the first cohort of brain-focused psychiatrists began to emerge in American psychiatry. Though they were far outnumbered by the Freudians, members of organizations like the Society of Biological Psychiatry revived the brain-focused studies of their German forebears. But they did not limit themselves to the examination of postmortem specimens; they also trolled for clues in the bodily fluids of living patients—the blood, cerebral spinal fluid, and urine. The new generation of biological psychiatrists believed that somewhere in this organic soup they would find their Holy Grail: a biological marker for mental illness.

Just as John Cade believed that mania was produced by a metabolic toxin, the biological psychiatrists hypothesized that mental illness might be caused by some pathogenic organic compound aberrantly produced by the body—a compound presumably detectable through laboratory tests. The inspiration for this hypothesis was a metabolic disorder known as phenylketonuria (PKU), a condition caused by a genetic mutation that prevents the liver from metabolizing phenylalanine, an essential amino acid. The faulty metabolism in individuals with PKU produces an accumulation of a substance known as *phenylketone*. Too much phenylketone interferes with the brain's development and leads to intellectual disability and behavioral problems. Thus, phenylketone serves as a biomarker for PKU: If physicians detect the compound in a patient's blood or urine, it indicates he probably has the disorder, since people without this condition have extremely low levels of phenylketone.

In the mid-1960s, biological psychiatrists began searching for a biomarker by comparing the urine of mentally ill patients and healthy individuals with a new technique called chromatography. Chromatography uses a special chemical-sensitive paper that turns a different color for each distinct compound it comes into contact with. If you place a drop of urine from a healthy person onto one strip of paper and a drop of urine from an ill person onto another and then compare the colors on each strip, you can identify differences in the types and amounts of the urine's chemical constituents—and these differences might reflect the biochemical by-products of the illness.

In 1968, the biological psychiatrists' chromatographic efforts paid off with a sensational breakthrough. Researchers at the

University of California at San Francisco discovered that the urine of schizophrenia patients produced a color that did not appear in the urine of healthy individuals—a "mauve spot." Enthusiasm among biological psychiatrists only increased when another group of researchers discovered in the urine of schizophrenics the existence of a separate "pink spot." Many believed that psychiatry was on the verge of a new era, when psychiatrists could discern the entire rainbow of mental ill-nesses merely by instructing patients to pee on a scrap of paper.

Unfortunately, this urine-fueled optimism was short-lived. When other scientists attempted to replicate these wondrous findings, they uncovered a rather mundane explanation for the mauve and pink spots. It seemed that the putative biomark-ers were not by-products of the schizophrenia itself, but by-prod-ucts of antipsychotic drugs and caffeine. The schizophrenic patients who participated in the chromatography studies were (quite sensibly) being treated with antipsychotic medications and—since there was not much else to do in a mental ward—they tended to drink a lot of coffee and tea. In other words, the urine tests detected schizophrenia by identifying individu-als taking schizophrenia drugs and consuming caffeinated beverages.

While the search for biomarkers in the 1960s and '70s ulti-mately failed to produce anything useful, at least it was driven by hypotheses that posited physiological dysfunction as the source of mental illness, rather than sexual conflicts or "refrig-erator mothers." Eventually biological psychiatrists broadened their search for the diagnostic Holy Grail beyond the bodily fluids. They turned instead to the substance of the brain itself. But since the organ was encased within impenetrable bone and sheathed in layers of membranes, and couldn't be studied without risking damage, how could they hope to peer into the mystifying dynamics of the living brain?

Throwing Open the Doorways to the Mind

Since so little was learned about mental illness from the visual inspection of cadaver brains in the nineteenth and early twentieth centuries, psychiatrists suspected that any neural signatures associated with mental disorders must be much more subtle than the readily identifiable abnormalities resulting from strokes, age-related dementias, tumors, and traumatic brain injuries. What was needed was some way to peer inside the head to see the brain's structure, composition, and function.

The invention of X-rays by Wilhelm Roentgen in 1895 seemed, at first, the longed-for technological breakthrough. X-rays aided the diagnosis of cancer, pneumonia, and broken bones... but when early radiographs were taken of the head, all they showed was the vague outline of the skull and brain. Roentgen's rays could detect skull fractures, penetrating brain injuries, or large brain tumors, but not much else of use to biologically minded psychiatrists.

If psychiatrists were to have any hope of detecting physical evidence of mental illness in the living brain, they would need an imaging technology that revealed the fine architecture of the brain in discernible detail or, even better, somehow disclosed the actual activity of the brain. In the 1960s, this seemed an impossible dream. When the breakthrough finally came, the funding that enabled it came from a most surprising source: the Beatles.

In the early 1970s, the EMI corporation was primarily a record company, but they did have a small electronics division, as reflected in their unabbreviated name: Electric and Musical Industries. EMI's music division was raking in enormous profits from the phenomenal success of the Beatles, the world's most popular band. Flush with cash, EMI decided to take a chance on a highly risky and expensive project in its electronics division. The EMI engineers were trying to combine X-rays from multiple angles in order to produce three-dimensional images of objects. Surmounting technical obstacles using profits from "I Want to Hold Your Hand" and "With a Little Help from My Friends," EMI engineers created a radiographic technology that obtained images of the body that were far more comprehensive and detailed than anything in medical imaging. Even better, the resulting procedure was not invasive and elicited no physical discomfort in the patients. EMI's new technology became known as *computed axial tomography*—more commonly referred to as the CAT scan.

The first study of mental illness using the CAT scan was published in 1976 by Eve Johnstone, a British psychiatrist, and it contained an astounding finding: the very first physical abnormality in the brain associated with one of the three flagship mental illnesses. Johnstone found that the brains of schizophrenic patients had enlarged lateral ventricles, a pair of chambers deep within the brain that contain the cerebrospinal fluid that nourishes and cleanses the brain. Psychiatrists were thunderstruck. Ventricular enlargement was already known to occur in neurodegenerative diseases like Alzheimer's when the brain structures surrounding the ventricles began to atrophy, so psychiatrists naturally inferred that the ventricular enlargement in schizophrenic brains was due to atrophy from some unknown process. This landmark finding was promptly replicated by an American psychiatrist, Daniel Weinberger at the NIMH.

Before the shock waves from the first psychiatric CAT scans had begun to subside, another brain-imaging marvel arrived that was even better suited for studying mental disorders: magnetic resonance imaging (MRI). MRI used a revolutionary new technology that enveloped a person within a powerful magnet and measured the radio waves emitted by organic molecules of the body when they were excited by the magnetic field. MRI was used to image the brain for the first time in 1981. Whereas the

Normal Control   Patient with Schizophrenia

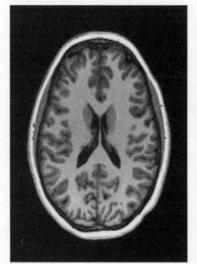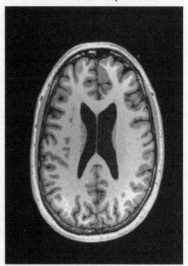

MRI in the axial view (looking down through the top of the head) of a patient with schizophrenia on reader's right and a healthy volunteer on the left. The lateral ventricles are the dark butterfly-shaped structure in the middle of the brain. (Courtesy of Dr. Daniel R. Weinberger, MD, National Institute of Mental Health)

CAT scan enabled psychiatric researchers to peek through a keyhole at brain abnormalities, MRI thrust the door wide open. MRI technology was able to produce vivid three-dimensional images of the brain in unprecedented clarity. The MRI could even be adjusted to show different types of tissue, including gray matter, white matter, and cerebral fluid; it could identify fat and water content; and it could even measure the flow of blood within the brain. Best of all, MRI was completely harmless— unlike CAT scans, which used ionizing radiation that could accumulate over time and potentially pose a health risk.

By the end of the 1980s, the MRI had replaced CAT scans as the primary instrument of psychiatric research. Other applications of MRI technology were also developed in the '80s, including magnetic resonance spectroscopy (MRS, measuring the chemical composition of brain tissue), functional magnetic resonance imaging (fMRI, measuring brain activity rather than brain structure), and diffusion tensor imaging (DTI, measuring the long tracts that carry signals between neurons).

The brain imaging bonanza of the '80s wasn't limited to magnetic technologies. The decade also witnessed the refinement of positron emission tomography (PET), a technology that can measure the brain's chemistry and metabolism. While PET provides only a hazy picture of brain *structure*—compared to the fine spatial resolution afforded by MRI—PET measures the brain's chemical and metabolic *activity* in quantitative detail. Perhaps anticipating the use of PET scans by psychiatrists, James Robertson, the engineer who carried out the very

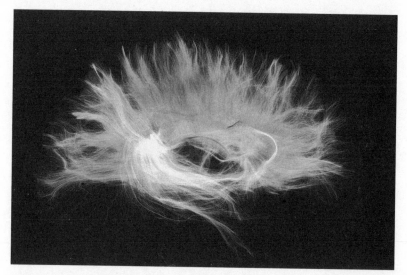

Diffusion Tensor Image of the brain presented in the sagittal plane (looking sideways at the head with the front on the right side of picture and the back on the left side). The white matter fibers that connect neurons in the brain into circuits are depicted removed from the matrix of gray matter, cerebrospinal fluid, and blood vessels. (Shenton et al./*Brain Imaging and Behavior*, 2012; vol. 6, issue 2; image by Inga Koerte and Marc Muehlmann)

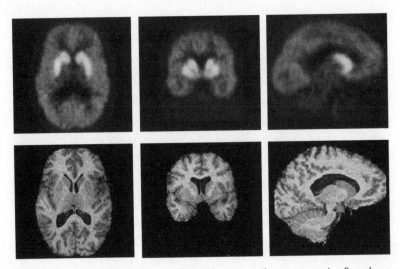

PET scan images (top row) and MRI images (bottom row) of patients presented in three planes of view. Left column is the axial plane (looking at brain through the top of the head), middle column is the coronal plane (looking at brain through the face), and the right column is the sagittal plane (looking at brain through the side of the head). The PET scan is of a radiotracer (biologic dye) that binds to dopamine receptors in the brain which are concentrated in the bright structures (basal ganglia) in the brain's interior and more diffusely in the surrounding cerebral cortex. The MRI that shows the brain's structure, highlighting the gray and white matter and the ventricles and subarachnoid space containing cerebrospinal fluid (black), is used in combination with PET scans to determine the anatomic locations where the radiotracer has bound. (Abi-Dargham A. et al./*Journal of Cerebral Blood Flow & Metabolism*, 2000; 20:225–43. Reproduced with permission.)

first PET scans at the Brookhaven National Laboratory, nicknamed the PET scanner the "head-shrinker."

As a result of these magnificent new imaging technologies, by the end of the twentieth century psychiatrists could finally examine the brain of a living person in all its exquisite splendor: They could view brain structures to a spatial resolution of less than a millimeter, trace brain activity to a temporal resolution of less than a millisecond, and even identify the chemical composition of brain structures—all without any danger or discomfort to the patient.

The venerable dream of biological psychiatry is starting to be fulfilled: after studying hundreds of thousands of people with virtually every mental disorder in the *DSM*, researchers have begun identifying a variety of brain abnormalities associated with mental illness. In the brains of schizophrenic patients, structural MRI studies have revealed that the hippocampus is smaller than in healthy brains; functional MRI studies have shown decreased metabolism in frontal cortex circuits during problem-solving tasks; and MRI studies have found increased levels of the neurotransmitter glutamate in the hippocampus and frontal cortex. In addition, PET studies have shown that a neural circuit involved in focusing attention (the mesolimbic pathway) releases excessive amounts of dopamine in schizophrenic brains, distorting the patients' perceptions of their environments. We've also learned that schizophrenic brains exhibit a progressive decline in the amount of gray matter in their cerebral cortex over the course of the illness, reflecting a reduction in the number of neural synapses. (Gray matter is brain tissue that contains the bodies of neurons and their synapses. White matter, on the other hand, consists of the axons, or wires, which connect neurons to one another.) In other words, if schizophrenics are not treated, their brains get smaller and smaller.

There have been similar neural revelations about other mental disorders. In 1997, Helen Mayberg, a neurologist at Emory University, used PET imaging to examine the brains of depressed patients and made a startling discovery: Their subgenual cingulate gyrus, a small structure deep in the front part of the brain, was hyperactive. And that wasn't all—when these patients were treated with antidepressant medication, the excessive activity in their subgenual cingulate gyrus was reduced to that of healthy subjects. Mayberg's finding led directly to a new type of therapy for individuals suffering from very severe depression who did not respond to medication: *deep brain stimulation*. During DBS, electrodes are directly implanted into a patient's brain in the region of the subgenual cingulate gyrus to reduce the firing of neurons causing the hyperactivity.

Imaging studies have also unveiled some very interesting details regarding suicide. The vast majority of people who commit suicide suffer from a mental illness, with depression being the most common. Yet, not everyone who suffers from depression becomes suicidal. This prompted researchers to ask if there might be some difference in the brains of those depressed individuals who *do* decide to take their own lives. Subsequent studies have revealed that their brains have an increase in a particular kind of serotonin receptor (5-HT1A) located in a part of the brain stem known as the dorsal raphe. The increase in dorsal raphe serotonin receptors was first identified in the postmortem brains of individuals who had committed suicide, and then confirmed in living patients using PET imaging.

PET and fMRI studies have also demonstrated that patients with anxiety disorders have an overactive amygdala in their brains. The amygdala is a small almond-shaped structure on the inner surface of the temporal lobe that plays a critical role in our emotional reaction to events. Research has shown that when pictures that provoke emotional reactions are presented to an individual with an anxiety disorder, his amygdala tends to produce an exaggerated response compared to the brains of healthy patients. (We will learn more about the amygdala's crucial role in mental illness in the next chapter.)

The brains of infants suffering from autism evince distinct structural signatures that appear during the first twenty-four months of life as the illness first takes hold. The white matter develops differently in autistic brains, an abnormality detectable as early as six months of age, which seems to mean that the connections between certain brain cells are not getting properly established in autistic children. In addition, the cerebral cortex of autistic infants expands excessively in the second year of life, possibly due to the failure of the mechanism by which the proliferation of synaptic connections is regulated.

But sometimes understanding the brain requires more than just gazing at pictures—it requires conducting actual experiments on the gritty, wet reality of neural circuits, cells, and molecules. From the 1900s to the 1970s, very few psychiatrists spent any effort at all trying to understand the physiological operations of the brain directly in humans or by using animals as was done in the other medical specialties. After all, most psychiatrists during this long era of stagnation believed that mental illness was ultimately a psychodynamic or social issue. But a lone American psychoanalyst decided that the path to understanding the mind ran straight through the fissures of the brain.

The Other Psychiatrist from Vienna

Eric Kandel was born in 1929 in Vienna, Austria, not far from the home of seventy-three-year-old Sigmund Freud. In 1939, because of the *Anschluss*, Kandel's family fled to Brooklyn, New York, as Freud's family fled to London. Kandel was profoundly affected by his childhood experience, watching a city of friendly neighbors turn into a mob of hateful racists. Consequently he entered Harvard with the intent to study European history and literature in order to understand the social forces that produced such a malevolent transformation in his countrymen.

While at Harvard, he began dating a young woman named Anna Kris. One day she introduced him to her parents, Ernst and Marianne Kris, eminent psychoanalysts who had been members of Freud's inner circle in Vienna before immigrating to the United States. When Ernst asked the young Kandel about his academic goals, Kandel replied that he was studying history in order to make sense of anti-Semitism. Ernst shook his head and told Kandel that if he wanted to understand human nature, he should not study history—he should study psychoanalysis.

On the recommendation of his girlfriend's father, Kandel read Freud for the first time. It was a revelation. While Kandel eventually lost touch with Anna, her father's influence endured. Some forty years later, in his Nobel Prize address, Kandel recalled, "I was converted to the view that psychoanalysis offered a fascinating new approach—perhaps the only approach—to understanding the mind, including the irrational nature of motivation and unconscious and conscious memory."

After graduating from Harvard in 1952, Kandel entered New York University Medical School intending to become a psychoanalyst. But in his senior year, he made a decision that set him apart from most would-be shrinks: He decided that if he truly wanted to understand Freudian theory, he needed to study the brain. Unfortunately, nobody on the faculty at NYU actually did that. So during a six-month elective period, when most medical students were doing rotations on clinical services, Kandel ventured uptown to the laboratory of Harry Grundfest, an accomplished neurobiologist at Columbia University.

Kandel asked Grundfest if he might assist on research in his lab. Grundfest inquired what Kandel was interested in studying. Kandel replied, "I want to find out where the ego, id, and superego are located." At first, Grundfest could barely contain his laughter, but then he gave the ambitious young medical student some sober advice: "If you want to understand the brain, then you're going to have to study it one nerve cell at a time."

Kandel spent the next six months in Grundfest's lab learning how to record the electrical activity of individual neurons.

For an aspiring psychiatrist, this was a peculiar and question-able endeavor—akin to an economics student trying to under-stand economic theory by learning how the Bank of England printed banknotes. But as Kandel gradually mastered the use of microelectrodes and oscilloscopes, he came to believe that Grundfest was right: Studying nerve cells was the royal road to understanding human behavior.

By the time Kandel left the Columbia lab he had become convinced that the secrets of mental illness lay hidden within neural circuitry. Even so, he still maintained an abiding belief that psychoanalysis offered the best intellectual framework for understanding these secrets. In 1960, he began his psychiatric residency at the Freud-dominated Massachusetts Mental Health Center, where he underwent his own psychoanalysis. By 1965, Kandel had become a rare bird indeed: a fully accred-ited psychoanalytical psychiatrist who was also well trained in the techniques of neural research—simultaneously a psycho-dynamic psychiatrist and a biological psychiatrist. So what kind of a career would a young physician with such seemingly paradoxical interests pursue?

Kandel decided to study memory, since the neurotic con-flicts so central to the Freudian theory of mental illness were predicated upon memories of emotionally charged experiences. If he could understand how memories worked, he felt he would understand the fundamental mechanism behind the formation of neurotic conflicts, which were the basis of mental illness. But rather than probe patients' memories through word associa-tions, dream analysis, and talk therapy, Kandel took as his pro-fessional project something no psychiatrist had ever attempted before: the elucidation of the biological basis of memory.

His prospects were far from encouraging. In the mid-1960s, virtually nothing was known about the cellular mecha-nisms involved with memory. The nascent field of neuroscience was hardly a guide, since it hadn't yet coalesced into a coherent discipline. No medical schools boasted departments of neuroscience, and the Society for Neuroscience, the first professional organization representing this field, was not founded until 1969. If Kandel wanted to unravel the mysterious neural tapestry of memory, he would have to do it on his own.

Kandel guessed that the formation of memories must rely on modifications in the synaptic connections between neurons. But there was not yet any known way to study synaptic activity in humans. He considered investigating synapses in rodents, a common lab animal used in behavioral studies in the 1960s, but even the rat brain was too sophisticated to use as a starting point. Kandel realized he needed a much simpler organism—a creature whose brain was less complicated than a rat's, but still large enough that he could analyze the cellular and molecular processes of its neurons. After a long search, he finally hit upon the perfect beast: the California sea slug, *Aplysia californica.*

This marine mollusk possesses an extremely simple nervous system consisting of just 20,000 neurons, compared to about 100 billion in the human brain. At the same time, the cell bodies of the sea slug's neurons are easily visible and extremely large by anatomical standards: about 1 millimeter in diameter, compared to 0.1 millimeter in humans. While a sea slug's memories are obviously much different from a human's, Kandel hoped that by studying the small invertebrate he might discover the physiological mechanisms by which any animal's memories were formed. His reasoning was based upon the evolutionary theory of conservation: Since memory was both biologically complex and essential for life, once the basic cellular mechanisms of memory evolved in a very ancient species, the same mechanisms were probably conserved in the neurons of all its varied descendents. In other words, Kandel speculated that the cellular processes for encoding memories were the same for sea slugs, lizards, rats—and humans.

Kandel toiled in his laboratory at New York University,

painstakingly subjecting the sea slugs to a series of conditioned learning experiments of the same general sort that Ivan Pavlov once administered to salivating dogs. Kandel studied simple reflexes, such as the withdrawal of the sea slug's gill when something touched its siphon, and discovered that these reflexes could be modified through experience. For example, after gently touching the slug's siphon, he zapped the slug's tail with an electrical jolt, which caused the slug to retract its gill much more powerfully. Eventually, the slug retracted its gill powerfully from the gentle touch alone, which showed the creature knew that the touch signaled an impending jolt—the slug *remembered* the previous jolts.

After the sea slug demonstrated a new memory, Kandel cut the slimy creature open and painstakingly examined its neurons for any structural or chemical changes that might make up the biological signature of the slug's memory. This was quite likely the very first time that a psychiatrist used a nonhuman creature to study brain functions related to human mental activities, a method of experimental investigation that scientists refer to as an "animal model." While animal models had long been common in other fields of medicine, most psychiatrists had assumed it was not possible to emulate the seemingly uniquely human mental states in an animal—especially not in a primitive invertebrate.

Most psychiatrists paid little attention to Kandel's research, and those who did usually considered it interesting but irrelevant to clinical psychiatry. What could sea snails possibly have in common with an orally fixated person with a passive dependent personality or the superego rigidity of the obsessive-compulsive patient? How could identifying a snail's memory of an air puff to its gill help psychiatrists resolve unconscious conflicts or better understand the patient's transference to their therapist?

But Kandel persisted. After years of research on the giant neurons of the *Aplysia californica*, Kandel made a profound discovery. As Kandel explained to me, "I began to see what happens when you produce a short-term memory and, even more interesting, when you convert a short-term memory to a long-term one. Short-term memory involves transient changes in the activation of connections between nerve cells. There is no anatomical change. Long-term memory, on the other hand, involves enduring structural changes from the growth of new synaptic connections. I finally began to understand how the brain changes because of experience." Kandel's discovery of the divergent biological mechanisms of short-term and long-term memory remains one of the most important foundational principles of modern neuroscience.

In addition to his groundbreaking work on memory, Kandel also made an impressive series of discoveries that enhanced our understanding of anxiety disorders, schizophrenia, addiction, and aging. For example, Kandel's lab isolated a gene called RbAp48 that produces a protein involved in memory formation in the hippocampus. Kandel discovered that this gene is expressed less and less as we age, suggesting that treatments that sustain or increase the gene's activity could potentially reduce age-related memory loss. As our expected lifespan continues to increase, RbAp48 might just hold the key to preserving our memories in our ever-lengthening golden years.

Kandel's greatest contribution to psychiatry, though, may not have been any single neurobiological discovery, but his cumulative influence over psychiatry's direction. As a new generation of psychiatrists came of age in the 1970s and witnessed the therapeutic effects of psychopharmaceuticals and the new images of living brains, they began to believe there was more to mental illness than psychodynamics. The brain beckoned as an unopened treasure chest of insights and therapies—but how to unlock the mysteries of this mysterious organ? There was little psychiatric scholarship on the brain itself, and even less research on the cellular and molecular mechanisms of the brain. The few dedicated brain researchers tended to focus on relatively tractable functions like vision, sensation, and movement. Very few possessed the audacity (or foolishness) to tackle the higher mental functions underpinning human behavior... and Eric Kandel was the first of these few.

Before Kandel, very few psychiatric researchers used the research methodologies routinely used in other areas of biomedical research, and those who did had to seek training in the laboratories of scientists outside psychiatry, as did Kandel. Kandel showed how brain functions could be studied at the cellular and molecular levels in a way that could inform our understanding of the operation of the mind. By the late '70s, Kandel had emerged as *the* iconic role model of the psychiatric neuroscientist, inspiring a new generation of young research psychiatrists to incorporate brain science into their own careers.

Psychiatrists Steven Hyman (former NIMH director and Harvard provost) and Eric Nestler (chair of neuroscience at Mt. Sinai School of Medicine) were both the intellectual progeny of Kandel. In 1993, they published a seminal volume entitled *The Molecular Foundations of Psychiatry* that transformed the way psychiatrists thought about their own field. Inspired by Kandel's three decades of pioneering research, Hyman and Nestler's book described how basic neuroscience methods could be applied to the study of mental illness.

Ken Davis (CEO and dean of Mt. Sinai Medical Center) was another early psychiatric neuroscientist influenced by Kandel. Davis developed treatments based on the cholinergic theory of Alzheimer's disease, which directly led to the most popular Alzheimer's medications, including Aricept and Reminyl. Tom Insel (current director of NIMH) decided to shift his research career in midstream from clinical psychiatry to basic neuroscience—a gutsy move at the time—because of Kandel's visionary research.

The generation of psychiatric neuroscientists that followed forged further inroads into the mysterious workings of the brain. Karl Deisseroth, a Stanford psychiatrist trained in molecular biology and biophysics, devised disruptively innovative techniques (optogenetics and clarity) to elucidate brain structure and function, which have won him widespread acclaim. In every way he is heir to Kandel's legacy—a clinically attuned psychiatrist who continues to see patients and a world-class neuroscientist—including the fact that he is the leading candidate to be the next psychiatrist to win the Nobel Prize.

Kandel's long, solitary journey in search of memory ultimately led to widespread acclaim. In 1983, he received the Lasker Award for Basic Science. In 1988, he was awarded the

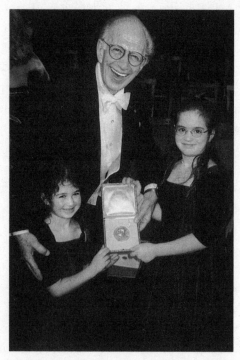

Eric Kandel with grandchildren at the Nobel ceremony in Stockholm, Sweden, December 10, 2000. (Photograph by Tomas Hökfelt, from Eric Kandel's personal collection)

National Medal of Science. And in 2000 he received the greatest accolade available to any researcher, the Nobel Prize in Physiology and Medicine. Today, young psychiatrists take brain research for granted. MD-PhDs—researchers trained as both physicians and scientists—are now as common in psychiatry as in any other medical discipline. And while Kandel was only the second psychiatrist to receive the Nobel (Julius Wagner-Jauregg received the first for his malaria cure, and Moniz was a neurologist), after his trailblazing career I don't think we will be waiting long for a third.

Reforming Talk Therapy

As dramatic breakthroughs in psychopharmacology, neuroimaging, and neuroscience strengthened biological psychiatry and fomented a brain revolution, the science of psychodynamic psychiatry was advancing on a parallel track. The 1960s saw the first meaningful advances in what was still psychiatry's principal mode of treatment: talk therapy.

Ever since Freud first established the ground rules for psychotherapy at the beginning of the twentieth century, psychoanalysis had been king of the consulting room. For generations, the public associated a visit to a shrink with reclining on a couch or comfortable chair and unloading all the neurotic minutiae of their lives in an hour-long session, a characterization frequently depicted in the early films of Woody Allen. The unquestioned Freudian rules of engagement required the doctor to remain remote and impersonal; expressions of emotion and empathy were forbidden. Psychiatrists as recently as the 1990s were still being trained to stay aloof, deflecting a patient's questions with questions of their own. Family photographs, diplomas, and any other personal emblems were kept out of the shrink's office to maintain the illusion of impenetrable anonymity.

When change finally came to this ossified mode of talk therapy, it was at the hands of a disillusioned psychoanalyst. Many of the most disruptive challenges to psychoanalysis were instigated by onetime Freudians: ex-psychoanalyst Robert Spitzer eliminated neurosis as a psychiatric diagnosis in the 1970s; ex-psychoanalyst Nathan Kline pioneered psychopharmacological treatments in the 1960s; and in a moment akin to Martin Luther nailing his ninety-five theses to the Wittenberg church door, psychoanalyst Tim Beck committed professional heresy when he declared there was another means by which to effect therapeutic change, through psychotherapy rather than psychoanalysis.

Aaron "Tim" Beck was born in Rhode Island in 1921, the son of Russian Jewish immigrants. After graduating from the Yale University School of Medicine, Beck became a psychiatrist and embraced the prevailing theory of the age. In 1958 he wrote to a colleague, "I have come to the conclusion that there is one conceptual system that is peculiarly suitable for the needs of the medical student and physician-to-be: Psychoanalysis."

Beck was so completely convinced that psychoanalytic theory represented the correct way to think about mental illness that he wanted to prove to skeptics that scientific research could test psychoanalytic theory. In 1959, he decided to carry out an experiment designed to validate a psychoanalytic theory of depression known as "inverted hostility." This theory held that a person suffering from depression was angry at someone else (frequently a parent) but was unconsciously redirecting this anger toward himself. As an example, imagine that your significant other leaves you for someone more attractive; inverted hostility suggested that rather than expressing anger toward your ex, you'd say he had done nothing wrong at all, but you'd feel angry at yourself for having driven him away, which would express itself as sadness and paralysis.

One of the predictions of inverted hostility theory was that depressed individuals would feel better about themselves after a failure, while they should feel worse about themselves after a success. This convoluted logic was predicated on the idea that since a depressed individual was angry at herself (the "inverted hostility"), she did not deserve success and would want to punish herself, and therefore would feel satisfaction when the object of her hostility (herself) failed at a task. Beck rigged a card-sorting test so that he could control whether his subjects succeeded or failed, and then measured their self-esteem afterward. To his astonishment, his results showed the exact opposite of what he had expected: When depressed individuals were allowed to attain success at sorting cards, they felt much better; but when they were forced to fail, they felt worse. "After that, I became suspicious that the entire theory was wrong," Beck says.

With his Freudian blinders loosened, Beck began paying careful attention to the precise nature of his depressed patients' cognition. "Psychoanalytic theory insisted that depressed people should have excessive hostility in their dreams because of their inverted hostility. But when you looked at the content of their dreams, they actually had *less* hostility in them than normal people did," Beck explains. Instead, Beck noticed that his depressed patients experienced streams of distorted thoughts that seemed to spontaneously surge forth. These "automatic thoughts," as Beck labeled them, had nothing to do with anger but instead reflected "illogical ideas about themselves and the world they lived in." A middle-aged woman who was attractive and accomplished might relentlessly describe herself as incompetent. Beck believed that this negativism rendered her perpetually distracted and cheerless and eventually led to her being depressed. This was a radical revision of psychiatry's conception of depression—instead of characterizing depression as an *anger* disorder, he characterized it as a *cognitive* disorder.

Redefining the nature of depression was already the kind of thing that would have got Beck excommunicated by Freud had he still been alive, but then he made another heretical discovery: When he stopped trying to get patients to understand their buried neurotic conflicts and instead used talk therapy to help his patients *correct* their illogical thoughts and *change* their self-defeating perceptions, they became happier and more productive. Even more astonishing, these psychic improvements took place at a much faster rate than under psychoanalysis—weeks, instead of months or years.

I asked Beck what it was like when he first saw the rapid effects of his new technique. "My patients would have ten or twelve sessions and then say, Terrific, you've helped me a lot, thanks, I'm ready to go handle this on my own, bye! My patient list shrunk down to zero because everybody was getting helped so fast. My department chair saw all my patients leaving and told me, 'You're not making it in private practice, why don't you try something else.'"

Rather than taking his chair's advice, Beck formalized his technique into an unprecedented method of psychotherapy that helped patients become aware of their distorted thoughts and taught them how to challenge these thoughts. Beck called this method cognitive-behavioral therapy, or CBT. Here's an abbreviated transcript of a conversation (from the book *Cognitive-Behavioral Therapy for Adult Attention Deficit Hyperactivity Disorder*) between a contemporary CBT therapist (T) and a patient with ADHD (P) who is afraid to sign up for a professionally necessary class because of his fears of what his ADHD will make him do:

T: What are your thoughts about the CPR course?
P: I've done a CPR course in the past and by the end it was hard to pay attention. I'd be worried I might make

some mistakes, especially when I'm working in a group with others.

T: Can you describe your apprehension in more detail, what specifically makes you feel that way?

P: These are the people who'd be coworkers, who I'd be working with and interacting with. I'd be worried about messing up in front of them.

T: And what would the consequence of that be?

P: We'd have to start over from the beginning and get retested because of me and I'd hold up the entire class.

T: Do you remember having had any experiences in your life in which the worries you've described—making mistakes in front of others or holding up a group— actually happened?

P: I don't know. It hasn't happened a lot. I've been able to avoid big embarrassments. In one CPR course I made a mistake during one of the team exercises. I was tired and I lost my focus.

T: When you realized you made a mistake, what thoughts did you have?

P: "What's wrong with me? Why can't I do this right?"

T: Okay. So there was a situation in your past that is similar to what you're concerned might happen in a longer CPR course. Recognizing you made a mistake is not a distorted thought. In this case, it was accurate—you made an error. However, it sounds as though the conclusions you drew that something was wrong with you may have been distorted. What was the reaction of your teammates when you had to redo the CPR sequence?

P: Nobody laughed, but I could see it in their faces that they were upset and that they were annoyed at me.

T: What did you see in their faces that was evidence that they were annoyed?

P: One lady rolled her eyes.

T: How long after the course do you think the lady thought about your mistake? Do you think she went home and told her family, "You won't believe what happened in CPR class today? This guy made a mistake during our final test?"

P: (Laughing) No. She probably didn't give it much thought.

Notice how the therapist listens carefully to what the patient says, and immediately responds to each assertion. The therapist is talking even more than the patient—a cardinal sin in psychoanalysis. Freud taught psychiatrists to remain remote and aloof, but the therapist in this exchange is engaged and supportive, and even injects some humor into his interactions with his patient. But the differences between Beck's CBT and traditional psychoanalysis ran even deeper.

Whereas psychoanalysis attempted to unearth impulses deeply buried in the unconscious, Beck was interested in the thoughts circling around and around in the waking consciousness. Whereas psychoanalysis attempted to uncover the historic motives behind troubling emotions, Beck scrutinized the immediate experience of a person's emotions. Whereas psychoanalysis was ultimately pessimistic, seeing neurotic conflict as the price for existing in a social world, Beck remained upbeat, suggesting that if people were willing to work hard on their problems, they could eliminate their neurotic tendencies.

CBT had an energizing and liberating effect on the field. Unlike psychoanalysis, which placed restrictions on the therapist's conduct and was undefined and open-ended, possibly lasting for years, CBT had a defined set of instructions for therapists, entailed a finite number of sessions, and established specific goals. CBT's therapeutic effects were soon validated in controlled experiments that compared the effects of CBT with a placebo and with different forms of psychoanalysis when treating depression, making CBT the first "evidence-based psychotherapy"—a form of talk therapy proven to work through a blind experiment. Since then, numerous studies have validated CBT's effectiveness as a treatment for many mental disorders, including anxiety disorders, obsessive-compulsive disorder, and ADHD.

The unexpected success of CBT opened the door to other kinds of evidence-based psychotherapy by showing that it was possible to treat patients more quickly and effectively than traditional psychoanalysis allowed. In the 1970s, two Yale faculty members created "interpersonal psychotherapy," a form of talk therapy for depressed patients that encourages patients to regain control of their moods and their lives. In the late 1980s, dialectical behavioral therapy, a highly focused form of psychotherapy for patients with borderline personality disorder, was created by a psychologist who suffered from the disorder herself. In 1991, two psychologists introduced motivational interviewing, a psychotherapeutic technique for treating addiction that fosters motivation.

Tim Beck's venture beyond the rigid precepts of psychoanalysis to explore the true nature of neurotic depression through experimentation enabled him to create a unique form of psychotherapy that improved the lives of millions of patients. By doing so, he demonstrated that rigorous science was not solely the purview of biological psychiatrists but could also be wielded to dramatic effect by psychodynamic psychiatrists.

Too Many Genes, Too Few Genes

By the mid-1980s, psychiatry was using more effective forms of psychotherapy, more effective psychopharmaceuticals, and more effective brain imaging. The field of neuroscience was rapidly gaining strength. There was growing acceptance among psychiatrists that people suffering from mental illness had something wrong in their brain—especially severe mental illnesses that previously required institutionalization, like schizophrenia, bipolar disorder, autism, and depression. But if something was wrong with your mentally ill brain, then where did this wrongness come from? Were you born to it? Or was it forged within you by your experiences in life? The answer turned out to be quite different than anyone expected.

The relationship between genes and mental illness did not interest the Freudians (who emphasized the role of childhood experiences) or the social psychiatrists (who emphasized the role of family and cultural environments). But in the early 1960s, a physician-scientist named Seymour Kety decided to investigate the genetic basis of mental illness, following up on the work of the German psychiatrist Franz Kallman. It had been known for centuries that mental illness ran in families—but families have many things in common that are not genetic, such as wealth, religion, and table manners, that come from a shared or common environment. The first question Kety attempted to answer seemed straightforward enough: Is schizophrenia primarily caused by genes or the environment?

Using Danish health registries, Kety found that the rate of schizophrenia in the population was about 1 percent, while the rate among individuals with at least one family member with schizophrenia was 10 percent. His data also revealed that if both your parents had schizophrenia, then you had a 50 percent chance of developing schizophrenia yourself. Similarly, if you had an *identical* twin with schizophrenia, then you also had a 50 percent chance of being schizophrenic, but if your *fraternal* twin had schizophrenia then your chance of being schizophrenic was only 10 percent. Thus, it seemed that the more genes you shared with a schizophrenic, the more likely you were to develop the disorder—though this correlation was clearly not perfect. After all, identical twins share 100 percent of the same genes, so if there was a "schizophrenia gene" in one twin, it should presumably be found in the other.

Citing this fact, many critics took Kety's finding as strong evidence that schizophrenia was primarily environmental, arguing that the greater incidence of schizophrenia within families with at least one schizophrenic member was due to an unhealthy domestic environment rather than anything genetic. To settle the question of schizophrenia's genetic basis, Kety started a new study. He identified individuals with schizophrenia who had been adopted at birth and examined the rates of schizophrenia among both adoptive and biological relatives. He found higher rates of schizophrenia in the biological relatives, but not in the adoptive families. He also found that children born to a mother with schizophrenia but reared in an adoptive family developed schizophrenia at the same rate as those reared by the biological mother with schizophrenia. These findings demonstrated that schizophrenia was at least partially due to one's genetic endowment, and not solely due to environmental factors like "double-binding mothers" or poverty.

Similar studies of other disorders quickly followed, showing that autism, schizophrenia, and bipolar disorder featured the highest heritability among mental disorders, while phobias, eating disorders, and personality disorders featured the lowest. Yet even though the epidemiologic studies carried out by Kety and other researchers seemed to demonstrate that a predisposition toward mental illnesses could be inherited, the findings posed a number of genetic puzzles. For one thing, even monozygotic twins—individuals with identical sets of genes—didn't always develop the same mental illness. Further complicating the picture was the fact that sometimes schizophrenia skipped entire generations, only to reemerge later in the family tree. And sometimes, schizophrenia appeared in individuals with no family history of the disease at all. All of this also held true with depression and bipolar disorder.

Another riddle was presented by the fact that individuals with schizophrenia or autism were less likely to form romantic relationships, marry, and have children compared to people without mental illnesses, yet the frequency of both disorders in the population remained relatively constant or increased over time. As the role of genetics gained prominence in biomedical research in the 1980s, psychiatrists became convinced that these strange patterns of inheritance would be explained once scientists discovered the fabled pot of gold at the end of the genetic rainbow: a specific gene (or gene mutation) that caused a specific mental illness.

Psychiatrists began searching for mental illness genes in unique, geographically isolated or founder populations like the Old Order Amish and among aboriginal peoples in Scandinavia, Iceland, and South Africa with all the fervor of miners headed for the Klondike gold rush. The first report of a mental illness gene came in 1988 from a team of British scientists led by geneticist Hugh Gurling. Gurling's team reported that they had "found the first concrete evidence for a genetic basis to schizophrenia" residing on chromosome 5. But Gurling's gene proved to be fool's gold: Other scientists could not replicate his finding with DNA from other schizophrenic patients. This reversal of fortune was to become a recurring and deeply frustrating pattern in psychiatric genetics.

By the 1990s, researchers had succeeded in identifying specific genes that caused illnesses like cystic fibrosis, Huntington's disease, and Rett syndrome, but psychiatric researchers were unable to pinpoint any specific gene associated with any mental illness. Psychiatrists began to experience an unsettling sense of déjà vu: More than a century earlier, using the cutting-edge technology of the era (the microscope), biological psychiatrists had been unable to identify any gross anatomical basis for mental illness, even though they were certain it must exist *somewhere*. And now it seemed to be happening again with genetics.

But in 2003, two game-changing events occurred. First, the Human Genome Project was completed, mapping the entire set of genes encoded in human DNA. This was soon followed by the invention of a stunning new genetic technique known as representational oligonucleotide microarray analysis (ROMA). Prior to ROMA, molecular geneticists analyzed genes by determining the sequence of nucleotides in a given gene to see if any nucleotide was missing or out of place (called single nucleotide polymorphisms, or SNPs). ROMA, in contrast, scanned a person's entire genome at once and tabulated the number of copies of a specified gene, revealing whether a person had too many copies of the gene or too few.

Michael Wigler, a biologist working at Cold Spring Harbor Laboratory, invented ROMA as a method to study cancer. But he quickly realized its implications for understanding mental illness, and with the help of geneticist Jonathan Sebat, Wigler began applying ROMA to the DNA of patients with autism, schizophrenia, and bipolar disorder. Before ROMA, the question that psychiatric geneticists asked was, "Which specific genes cause mental illness?" But ROMA reframed the question as: "Can too many (or too few) copies of a healthy gene cause mental illness?"

Using ROMA, Wigler and Sebat were able to examine a wide array of genes in mentally ill patients' DNA and compare them to the genes in healthy persons. They targeted genes that produced proteins essential to healthy brain functions, such as a gene that produced a protein forming part of a neurotransmitter receptor or guided the formation of neural connections. Their research paid off almost immediately. They found that mentally ill patients possessed the same brain-related genes in their DNA as their mentally healthy counterparts, but the patients possessed either *more copies* or *fewer copies* of these genes than healthy people. Wigler had discovered the genome's Goldilocks phenomenon: To have a healthy brain, not only did you need the right kind of genes, but you needed a "just right" number of these genes—neither too numerous nor too scarce.

Wigler's new methodology divulged other unexpected insights. While most genetic mutations in the DNA of patients with autism, schizophrenia, and bipolar disorder were specific to each illness, some genetic mutations were shared by two or more disorders, meaning that some manifestly different mental disorders shared common genetic factors. ROMA research also revealed a possible explanation for the sporadic nature of mental illness within families, such as how it skipped entire generations and sometimes appeared in only one identical twin: While a particular brain-related gene might get passed on to one's offspring (or appear in both twins), the number of copies of that gene could vary. Sometimes, copies of a gene were spontaneously created or deleted within the DNA of the sperm or egg cells. Even though twins shared 100 percent of the same *type* of genes, they didn't share 100 percent of the same *number of copies* of these genes.

Wigler's findings also provided a possible explanation for why older men and women are more likely to have children with mental conditions like autism or Down syndrome. Their egg and sperm cells have been genetically dividing and replicating for a longer period of time than in young parents, so they are more likely to introduce extra or fewer copies of genes into their children's DNA, since genetic replication errors accumulate over time and are more likely to occur than a mutation creating an entirely new gene.

As psychiatry progressed through the first decade of the twenty-first century, buoyed by the emergent technologies of brain imaging, neuroscience, and genetics as well as the proliferation of new pharmacological advances and psychotherapy, the once-stagnant field of psychiatry showed all the signs of a profession undergoing intellectual rejuvenation.

A New Kind of Psychiatry

When I first saw Jenn in 2005, the doctors couldn't figure out exactly what was wrong with her. A twenty-six-year-old woman born to an affluent family who had enjoyed a privileged upbringing, Jenn had attended private school in Manhattan and then a liberal arts college in Massachusetts, which is where her behavior first became problematic.

During her junior year, she became suspicious and guarded and stopped socializing with her friends. She began to exhibit severe mood swings. She was friendly and pleasant one day but volatile and nasty the next, often hurling caustic insults over minor provocations. Eventually her hostility and volatility became so disruptive that the college implored her parents to have her seen by a psychiatrist. They obeyed, taking her to a leading psychiatric facility in the Northeast, where she was promptly admitted. But when she was discharged she did not follow through with her aftercare appointments or take her prescribed medication. She relapsed repeatedly, leading to multiple hospitalizations, and with every relapse she got worse. What made her situation even more daunting was that each time she was admitted, the doctors seemed to give her a different diagnosis, including schizophrenia, schizoaffective disorder, and bipolar disorder.

I was asked to consult on Jenn when she was brought to New York Presbyterian Hospital–Columbia University Medical Center after a violent incident with her mother, prompted by Jenn's belief that her mother was trying to keep her from seeing her boyfriend. When I evaluated Jenn, her appearance was disheveled and her thinking seemed disorganized. She had been out of school for five years and was unemployed and living at home. She repeatedly voiced the conviction that a friend was trying to steal her boyfriend, and she explained to me that she and her boyfriend needed to immediately escape to New Mexico if they wanted to stay together.

After talking with Jenn's family, I learned that in reality the object of her affections had no interest in her. In fact, the young man had actually called Jenn's mother to complain that she was harassing him and threatening his real girlfriend. When Jenn's mother attempted to explain these facts to her daughter she became enraged and knocked her to the floor, prompting her current hospitalization.

During our conversation, Jenn seemed disengaged and distracted, behaviors commonly associated with schizophrenia—but they are associated with other conditions, too. Her false beliefs were not systematic delusions; they simply reflected unrealistic appraisals of her relationships with others. She exhibited a full range of emotions, and while her feelings were often intense and erratic, schizophrenics more typically exhibit emotions that are constricted and flat.

Although the diagnosis assigned to her upon admission was schizophrenia, my clinical intuition was telling me that something else was going on. But intuition must be supported by evidence, so I started gathering additional data. When I asked Jenn's parents about her early medical history, nothing much turned up—except for one fact. Her mother reported that Jenn was born prematurely and had a breech birth. That alone wouldn't account for her bizarre behaviors, but breech births and other forms of trauma during pregnancy and delivery are associated with a higher incidence of neurodevelopmental problems. A traumatic delivery can produce complications in the infant's brain, including a lack of oxygen, compression, or bleeding. In addition, due to an (Rh) incompatibility of blood types between her and her mother, she was born with anemia and required an immediate blood transfusion. As a consequence she had low Apgar scores (the ratings given by pediatricians to newborn babies to summarize their general physical status), indicating some birth distress, and she was kept in the neonatal intensive care unit for one week prior to going home.

I asked Jenn additional questions about her life and activities. She answered automatically with brief responses and seemed to be confused by the questions. She also exhibited limited concentration and poor memory. These marked cognitive impairments did not match the ones that usually occur in schizophrenia patients, who do not seem confused or forgetful as much as preoccupied and distracted, or engaged with imaginary stimuli. I began to wonder if Jenn's volatility and bizarre behavior may have been provoked by her environment rather than her genes.

I asked about her drinking and drug use. Eventually, she admitted she had used marijuana since the age of fourteen and cocaine since age sixteen, and while in college she smoked pot and snorted coke almost every day. A hypothesis began to take shape in my mind. I suspected she had sustained some mild form of brain injury from her birth trauma that caused a neurocognitive deficit, which was then exacerbated in adolescence by her heavy drug use, producing these quasi-psychotic behaviors. One piece of evidence supporting this diagnostic hypothesis was the fact that the antipsychotic drugs, which had previously been prescribed for her, did not have much of an effect on her condition.

I ordered tests that would help to assess my hypothesis. Neuropsychological test results revealed a significant discrepancy between her verbal and performance scores. With schizophrenia, verbal and performance scores tend to be similar even if lower overall than the population average. Performance scores are believed to be more sensitive to brain dysfunction than verbal scores, and the fact that Jenn's performance score was markedly lower than her verbal score suggested that she had some kind of acquired cognitive impairment. An MRI revealed markedly *asymmetric* enlargement of the lateral ventricles and subarachnoid space, an asymmetry more often associated with trauma or a vascular event (like a stroke) than mental illness (in schizophrenia the ventricular enlargement is more symmetrical). The social worker assisting me developed an extensive pedigree of Jenn's family using information provided by her parents that revealed a complete absence of mental illness in the family history. The only related condition in her biological relatives was substance abuse in some siblings and cousins.

I now felt confident about my diagnosis that her pathology was due to developmental injury and substance-induced toxicity. Her prior diagnoses of schizophrenia, schizoaffective disorder, and bipolar disorder had been reasonable guesses since in reality she suffered from a "phenocopy" of mental illness, meaning that she was exhibiting symptoms that mimicked a *DSM*-defined illness without suffering from the actual illness.

If Jenn had been admitted to a psychiatry ward thirty years ago when I started my training, she would have likely been committed to a long-term stay in a mental institution and almost certainly been given very powerful antipsychotic drugs that would have all but immobilized her. Or, she may have been subjected to months or years of psychoanalytic therapy exploring her childhood and especially her fraught relationship with her mother.

But in today's world of psychiatry, Jenn was swiftly discharged from the hospital and given intensive substance abuse treatment and rehabilitative cognitive and social therapies, along with a low dose of medication to help stabilize her during her course of treatment. The quality of her life gradually improved and today she is focused and engaged and expresses gratitude for the help she received in turning her life around. And while not living independently or professionally successful or married with children, she works part-time, lives peacefully with her mother, and has developed stable social relationships.

Jenn's modest recovery—one of a growing number of success stories—illustrates how clinical psychiatry has changed as a result of the brain revolution and the myriad scientific advances over the past decades. But there was one final breakthrough in the annals of psychiatry that helped shape the modern face of my profession—a breakthrough that may be the most overlooked and underappreciated discovery of them all.

Chapter 8

Soldier's Heart: The Mystery of Trauma

We don't want any damned psychiatrists making our boys sick.
— GENERAL JOHN SMITH, 1944

Military psychiatry is to psychiatry as military music is to music.
— CHAIM SHATAN, MD

Air Conditioner Anxiety

In 1972 I was living in a shabby brownstone near Dupont Circle in Washington, DC, a sketchy neighborhood back then. One morning as I was about to leave for my physiology class at George Washington University, I heard a hard knock on my apartment door. I opened it to find two young men staring straight at me with intense black eyes. I immediately recognized them as neighborhood toughs who often hung out on the street.

Without a word, they pushed me back into my apartment. The taller man pointed a large black pistol at me and growled, "Give us all your money!" My brain froze, like a computer encountering a file too large to open.

"Hey! I said *where is your goddamn money?*" he shouted, pressing the muzzle of the gun to my forehead.

"I don't have anything," I stammered. Wrong answer. The shorter man punched me in the face. The taller one smacked me on the side of my head with the gun. They shoved me into a chair. The shorter man began rummaging through my pock-

240

ets while the taller man went into my bedroom and began yanking out drawers and ransacking closets. After a few minutes of searching, they cursed with frustration; apart from the television, a stereo, and thirty dollars in my wallet, they weren't finding anything of value... but they hadn't checked my dresser.

Tucked away in the top drawer beneath a stack of underwear was a jewelry box containing my grandfather's Patek Philippe watch. I couldn't imagine losing it. He had given it to me before he died as a gift to his firstborn grandchild, and it was my most treasured possession.

"What else do you got? We know you got more!" the taller man shouted as he waved the gun in front of my face.

Then, a peculiar thing happened. My churning fear abruptly dissipated. My mind became calm and alert, even hyperalert. Time seemed to slow down. Clear thoughts formed in my mind, like orderly commands from air traffic control: "Obey and comply. Do what you need to do to avoid getting shot." Somehow, I believed that if I just kept my cool, I would escape with my life — and possibly the jewelry box, too.

"I don't have anything," I said calmly. "Take whatever you want, but I'm just a student, I don't have anything."

"What about your roommate?" the intruder spat, motioning toward the other bedroom. My roommate, a law student, was away at class.

"I don't think he has much, but take everything... anything you want." The taller man looked at me quizzically and tapped the gun against my shoulder a few times as if thinking. The two thugs looked at each other, then one abruptly yanked the thin gold chain off my neck, they hoisted up the television, stereo, and clock radio, and casually ambled out the front door.

At the time, the home invasion was the scariest experience of my life. You might expect that it shook me up, giving me nightmares or driving me to obsess about my personal safety. Surprisingly, no. After filing a useless report with the DC police, I replaced the appliances and went right on with my life. I didn't move to a new neighborhood. I didn't have bad dreams. I didn't ruminate over the intrusion. If I heard an unexpected knock on my door, I hopped up to answer it. I didn't even flinch when, months later, I saw one of them on the street on my way home. To be honest, I can no longer recall the details of the robbery very well at all, certainly no better than the details of *The Poseidon Adventure*, a suspenseful but unremarkable movie I saw that same year. Though I believe the gun was large and black, it could very well have been a small metal revolver. To my youthful mind the whole experience ended up seeming kind of thrilling, an adventure I had bravely endured.

Twelve years later, another dramatic event produced a very different reaction. I was living in an apartment on the fifteenth floor of a high-rise in Manhattan with my wife and three-year-old son. It was early October and I needed to remove the heavy air conditioner unit from my son's bedroom window and store it for the winter.

The unit was supported on the outside by a bracket screwed into the wall. I raised the window that pressed down onto the top of the air conditioner so I could lift the unit off the windowsill—a terrible mistake. The moment I lifted the window, the weight of the air conditioner tore the bracket from the outside wall.

The air conditioner began to tumble away from the building toward the usually busy sidewalk fifteen floors below. The machine seemed to hurtle down through the sky in a kind of cinematic slow motion. My life literally flashed before my eyes. All my dreams of a career in psychiatry, all my plans of raising a family, were plunging down with this mechanical meteor. I could do nothing but uselessly shriek, "Watch out!"

"Holy shit!" the doorman yelped as he frantically leapt away. Miraculously, the air conditioner smashed onto the pavement, not people. Pedestrians on both sides of the street all whipped their heads in unison toward the crashing sound of impact, but, thankfully, nobody was hurt.

I had escaped a high-stakes situation once again—but this time I was shaken to the depths of my being. I couldn't stop thinking about how stupid I was, how close I had come to hurting someone and ruining my life. I lost my appetite. I had trouble sleeping, and when I did I was plagued by graphic nightmares in which I painfully relived the air conditioner's fateful plunge. During the day I could not stop ruminating over the incident, playing it over and over in my mind like a video loop, each time reexperiencing my terror with vivid intensity. When I went into my son's room, I wouldn't go near the window, for the mere sight of it triggered disturbing feelings.

Even now, decades later, I can viscerally recall the fear and helplessness of those moments with little effort. In fact, just moments before I sat down to write about this incident, a Liberty Mutual Insurance commercial came on television. As the wistful song "Human" plays and Paul Giamatti's mellifluous voice expounds upon human frailty, a man accidentally drops an air conditioner out his window onto a neighbor's car. The ad is innocuous and witty, yet as I watched, I winced in fearful remembrance. Some part of me was instantly transported back to that terrifying moment watching my life plummet down fifteen stories...

These are all classic symptoms of one of the most unusual and controversial of mental illnesses: post-traumatic stress disorder (PTSD). One thing that sets PTSD apart from just about every other mental illness is that its origin is clear-cut and unequivocal: PTSD is caused by traumatic experience. Of the 265 diagnoses in the latest edition of the *DSM*, all are defined without any reference to causes, except for substance-use disorders and PTSD. While drug addiction is obviously due to an effect of the environment—the repeated administration of a chemical substance inducing neural changes—PTSD is the result of a psychological reaction to an event that produces lasting changes to a person's mental state and behavior. Before the event, a person appears mentally healthy. After the event, he is mentally wounded.

What is it about traumatic events that produce such intense and lasting effects? Why does trauma occur in some people and not in others? And how do we account for its seemingly unpredictable incidence—after all, it seems rather counterintuitive that dropping an air conditioner elicited PTSD-like effects, while a violent home invasion did not. During the latter episode I was assaulted and my life was in genuine danger; during the air conditioner's plunge, I never faced any physical hazard. Was there some critical factor that determined how my brain processed each event?

The unique nature and curious history of PTSD make it one of the most fascinating of all mental disorders. The story of PTSD encapsulates everything we've learned so far about psychiatry's tumultuous past: the history of diagnosis, the history of treatment, the discovery of the brain, the influence and rejection of psychoanalysis, and the slow evolution of society's attitude toward psychiatrists, from open derision to grudging respect. PTSD also represents one of the first times that psychiatry has achieved a reasonable understanding of how a mental disorder actually forms in the brain, even if our understanding is not yet complete.

The belated unriddling of PTSD commenced in a setting that was extremely inhospitable to the practice of psychiatry but extremely conducive to the generation of PTSD: the battlefield.

We Don't Have Time to Monkey Around with Guys Like That

In 1862, Acting Assistant Surgeon Jacob Mendez Da Costa was treating Union soldiers at Turner's Lane Hospital in Philadelphia, one of the largest military hospitals in the States. He had never seen such carnage, gaping bayonet wounds and ragged limbs blown off by cannon fire. In addition to observing the visible injuries, as he slowly worked his way through the casualties of the Peninsular campaign, Da Costa noticed that many soldiers seemed to exhibit unusual heart problems, particularly "a prompt and persistent tachycardia"—medical jargon for a racing heartbeat.

For example, Da Costa described a twenty-one-year-old private William C. of the 140th New York Volunteers, who sought treatment after suffering from diarrhea for three months and "had his attention drawn to his heart by attacks of palpitation, pain in the cardiac region, and difficulty in breathing at night." By the war's end, Da Costa had seen more than four hundred soldiers who exhibited the same peculiar and anomalous heart troubles, including many soldiers who had suffered no physical battlefield injuries at all. Da Costa attributed the condition to an "overactive heart damaged by ill use." He reported his observations in the 1867 publication by the United States Sanitary Commission and named this putative syndrome "irritable and exhausted soldier's heart." Da Costa suggested that *soldier's heart* could be treated with hospitalization and a tincture of digitalis, a drug that slows the heart rate.

Da Costa did not believe that the condition he had identified was in any way psychological, and no other Civil War physician made a connection between soldier's heart and the mental stress of warfare. In the official records of soldiers who refused to return to the front lines despite a lack of physical injury, the most common designations were "insanity" and "nostalgia"— that is, homesickness.

As bloody as the Civil War was, it paled in comparison to the mechanized horrors of World War I, the Great War. Heavy artillery rained down death from miles away. Machine guns ripped through entire platoons in seconds. Toxic gas scalded the skin and scorched the lungs. Incidents of soldier's heart increased dramatically and were anointed by British doctors with a new appellation: *shell shock*, based on the presumed link between the symptoms and the explosion of artillery shells.

Physicians observed that men suffering from shell shock not only exhibited the rapid heart rate first documented by Da Costa but also endured "profuse sweating, muscle tension, tremulousness, cramps, nausea, vomiting, diarrhea, and involuntary defecation and urination"—not to mention blood-curdling nightmares. In the memorable book *A War of Nerves,* by Ben Shepherd, British physician William Rivers describes a shell-shocked lieutenant rescued from a French battlefield:

> He had gone out to seek a fellow officer and found his body blown to pieces with head and limbs lying separated from his trunk.
>
> From that time he had been haunted at night by the vision of his dead and mutilated friend. When he slept he had nightmares in which his friend appeared, sometimes as he had seen him mangled in the field, sometimes in the still more terrifying aspect of one whose limbs and features had been eaten away by leprosy. The mutilated or leprous officer of the dream would come nearer and nearer until the patient suddenly awoke pouring with sweat and in a state of utmost terror.

Other symptoms of shell shock read like a blizzard of neurological dysfunction: bizarre gaits, paralyses, stammering, deafness, muteness, shaking, seizure-like fits, hallucinations, night terrors, and twitching. These traumatized soldiers were shown no sympathy by their superiors. Instead, shell-shocked soldiers were castigated as "gutless yellow-bellies" who couldn't stand up to the manly rigors of war. They were often punished by their officers—and occasionally executed for cowardice or desertion.

During World War I, psychiatrists were virtually absent from the military medical corps; military leaders did not want their soldiers exposed to the mental frailty and emotional weakness associated with psychiatry. The whole purpose of military training was to create a sense of invulnerability, a psychology of courage and heroism. Nothing could be more antithetical to that psychic hardening than the exploration and open expression of emotions encouraged by psychiatrists. At the same time, shell shock could not easily be ignored: roughly 10 percent of all soldiers serving in the Great War became emotionally disabled.

The first description of "wartime psychic trauma" in the medical literature was in a 1915 *Lancet* article written by two Cambridge University professors, psychologist Charles Myers and psychiatrist William Rivers. In the article, they adapted Freud's new psychoanalytic theory to explain shell shock in terms of repressed memories from childhood that became unrepressed by war trauma, thereby producing neurotic conflicts that intruded upon conscious awareness. To exorcise these neurotic memories, Rivers advocated the "power of the healer" (what Freud called transference) to lead the patient to a more tolerable understanding of his experiences.

Freud himself testified as an expert witness in a trial of Austrian physicians accused of mistreating *psychologically* wounded soldiers, and concluded that shell shock was indeed a bona fide disorder, distinct from common neuroses, but that it could be treated with psychoanalysis. Soon, psychiatrists applied other treatments to shell-shocked soldiers, including hypnosis and hearty encouragement, reportedly with favorable results. Still, there was nothing approaching consensus when it came to the nature or treatment of combat trauma.

While the horrors of the Great War were unprecedented, somehow World War II was even worse. Aerial bombardment, massive artillery, flamethrowers, grenades, claustrophobic submarines, and vicious landmines conspired with diabolical enhancements of World War I weaponry to produce even more frequent incidents of soldier's heart, now dubbed *battle fatigue, combat neurosis,* or *combat exhaustion.*

At first, the military believed that combat neurosis occurred only in cowards and psychological weaklings, and it began screening out recruits thought to possess deficiencies in their character; by these criteria over a million men were deemed unfit to fight because of perceived susceptibility to combat neurosis. But the military brass was forced to revise its thinking when the psychological casualty rate was still 10 percent of "mentally fit" soldiers. Moreover, some of these casualties were seasoned soldiers who had fought bravely.

The deluge of emotionally disabled soldiers compelled the military to reluctantly acknowledge the problem. In a startling reversal of attitude, the American army sought out the assistance of the shrinks who were just gaining prominence in civilian society. At the start of World War I, there were no psychiatrists in the military. At the start of World War II, the presence of psychiatrists in the American military was minimal: Out of the 1,000 members of the Army Medical Corps in 1939, only 35 were so-called neuropsychiatrists, the military's term for psychiatrists. (The term is misleading, since almost every neuropsychiatrist was a psychoanalyst who knew practically nothing about the neural architecture of the brain.) But as the war progressed and increasing numbers of soldiers came back physically whole but emotionally crippled, the military realized it needed to adjust its attitude toward psychiatry.

To combat the shortage of neuropsychiatrists, the military began to provide intensive psychiatric training to nonpsychiatric physicians. This training was authorized in an October 1943 letter from the Office of the Surgeon General addressing the "Early recognition and treatment of Neuropsychiatric Conditions in the Combat Zone," which may represent the first time the American military formally acknowledged the importance of "mental health" in active soldiers: "Because of the shortage of neuropsychiatrists, the attention of all medical officers is asked to attend to the responsibility for the mental as well as physical health of military personnel."

At the start of the war, the Office of the Surgeon General had two divisions: medicine and surgery. Now, because of need for more battlefield psychiatrists, a new division was added: neuropsychiatry. The first director of the new division was William C. Menninger, who would soon be assigned to produce the *Medical 203*, the direct forerunner of the *DSM-I*; he also became the first psychiatrist ever to hold the rank of brigadier general. In 1943, 600 physicians from other specialties were trained in neuropsychiatry and 400 neuropsychiatrists were directly recruited into the army. By the war's end, 2,400 army physicians had either been trained in neuropsychiatry or were neuropsychiatrists. A new role had been carved out for the psychiatrist: trauma physician.

Menninger's *Medical 203* included a detailed diagnosis of what was termed "combat exhaustion," but instead of viewing the condition as a single disorder, the *203* broke it down into a variety of possible neuroses stemming from wartime stress, including "hysterical neuroses," "anxiety neuroses," and "reactive depression neuroses." In 1945, the Department of Defense created a fifty-minute film that trained military physicians in the nuances of combat exhaustion. Despite its conspicuous psychoanalytic perspective, the training film takes a surprisingly progressive attitude toward the condition. It portrays a roomful of dubious military physicians who question the authenticity of combat exhaustion. One declares, "We're going to be dealing with soldiers who are really shot up, we won't have time to monkey around with guys like that." Another claims, "That soldier must have been a misfit from the start to break down." Then the instructor patiently explains to them that combat exhaustion can afflict even the most courageous and battle hardened of men and insists the condition is just as real and debilitating as a shrapnel wound.

Such a perspective was a striking turnaround for the military; it would have been simply unimaginable in World War I, when European and American militaries wanted nothing to do with psychiatry and shell-shocked soldiers were regarded as suffering from defects of character. Even so, many officers still scoffed at the idea of combat exhaustion and continued to dismiss soldier's heart as ordinary cowardice. During the Sicily campaign in 1943, General George Patton infamously visited wounded soldiers in an evacuation hospital when he came across a glassy-eyed soldier who didn't have any visible injuries. He asked the man what was wrong.

"Combat exhaustion," murmured the soldier.

Patton slapped him in the face and harangued him as a spineless malingerer. Afterwards he issued an order that anyone who claimed they could not fight because of combat exhaustion should be court-martialed. To the military's credit, Patton was reprimanded and ordered to apologize to the soldier by General Dwight D. Eisenhower.

Combat exhaustion turned out to be one of the few serious mental conditions that psychoanalytic treatment appeared to help. Psychoanalytical neuropsychiatrists encouraged trauma-

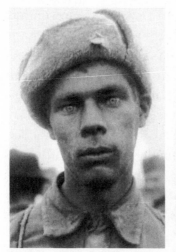 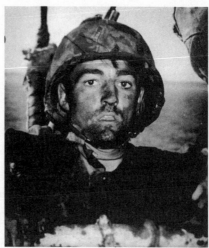

Russian soldier (left) and American soldier (right) exhibiting the "1,000-yard stare" characteristic of battle fatigue or combat exhaustion in World War II. (Right: U.S. Military, February 1944, National Archives 26-G-3394)

tized soldiers to acknowledge their feelings and express them, rather than keeping them bottled up as military training and masculine self-discipline dictated. They observed that soldiers who openly talked about their traumas tended to experience their battle fatigue less severely and recover faster. While the psychoanalytic reasoning behind this remedy was dubious—military neuropsychiatrists purported to be uncovering and alleviating buried neurotic conflicts—the effects were not, and today it is standard practice to provide empathic support to traumatized soldiers. Their apparent success in treating combat exhaustion with Freudian methods increased the self-confidence of military shrinks and motivated many of them to become enthusiastic proponents of psychoanalysis when they returned to civilian practice after the war, thereby aiding the Freudian conquest of American psychiatry.

Military neuropsychiatrists also learned that soldiers endure the stress of battle more for the comrades fighting next to them than for country or liberty, so if a traumatized soldier was sent home to recover—standard practice in the early years of World War II—this would cause him to feel guilt and shame for abandoning his comrades, which exacerbated rather than ameliorated his condition. So the army altered its practice. Instead of sending psychiatric casualties to military hospitals or returning them to the United States, it treated traumatized soldiers in field hospitals close to the front lines and then encouraged them to rejoin their units whenever possible.

Despite the small but meaningful advances in understanding the nature of psychological trauma, when World War II ended, psychiatry quickly lost interest. Combat exhaustion was not retained as a diagnosis but instead incorporated into a broad and vague category called "gross stress reaction" as part of *DSM-I* and then was omitted altogether from the *DSM-II*. Psychiatry's attention did not return to the psychological effects of trauma until the national nightmare that was Vietnam.

The Rap Group

Vietnam was the last American war to enlist soldiers through the draft. Unlike the world wars, the conflict in Southeast Asia was very unpopular. When the war escalated in the late 1960s, the government conducted a draft lottery to determine the order in which men would be sent to fight—and very possibly die—on the far side of the world. I was deferred from the draft due to my admission to medical school, but one of my classmates in college, a golden boy at our school—handsome, smart, athletic, class president—was drafted into the army as a lieutenant. Some years later I learned that he was killed in combat a few months after he landed in Vietnam.

The Vietnam War represented another major turning point in the American military's relationship with psychiatry. Yet again, a new war somehow found ways of becoming even more horrific than its horrific predecessors—sheets of napalm fire rained down from the sky and sloughed the skin off children, familiar objects like pushcarts and boxes of candy became improvised explosive devices, captured American soldiers were tortured for years on end. The Vietnam War produced more cases of combat trauma than World War II. Why? Two opinions are commonly expressed.

One view is that the Greatest Generation was stronger and more stoic than the Baby Boomers who fought in Vietnam. They came of age during the Great Depression, when boys were taught to "keep a stiff upper lip" and "suck it up," silently bearing their emotional pain. But there's another perspective I find more plausible. According to this explanation, veterans of World War II did sustain psychic consequences similar to those experienced by veterans of Vietnam, but society was simply not prepared to recognize the symptoms. In other words, the psychic damage to World War II veterans was hiding in plain sight and simply not recognized.

World War II was justifiably celebrated as a national triumph. Returning soldiers were celebrated as great victors, and Americans turned a blind eye to their psychic suffering, since emotional disability did not fit the prevailing notion of a valiant hero. Nobody was inclined to point out the changes and problems that veterans experienced upon returning home, for fear of being labeled unpatriotic. Even so, you can plainly see the signs of combat trauma in the popular culture of that era.

The Academy Award–winning 1946 film *The Best Years of Our Lives* portrayed the social readjustment challenges experienced by three servicemen returning from World War II. Each exhibits limited symptoms of PTSD. Fred is fired from his job after he loses his temper and hits a customer. Al has trouble relating to his wife and children; on his first night back from the war he wants to go to a bar to drink instead of staying home. A little-known documentary film produced by John Huston, the acclaimed director of *The African Queen*, and narrated by his father, Walter Huston, also depicted the psychological casualties of WWII. *Let There Be Light* follows seventy-five traumatized soldiers after they return home. "Twenty percent of our army casualties suffered psychoneurotic symptoms," the narrator intones, "a sense of impending disaster, hopelessness, fear, and isolation." The film was released in 1946 but was abruptly banned from distribution by the army on the purported grounds that it invaded the privacy of the soldiers involved. In reality, the army was worried about the film's potentially demoralizing effects on recruitment.

Another reason proposed for the increased incidence of combat trauma in Vietnam was the ambiguous motivation behind the war. In World War II, America was preemptively attacked at Pearl Harbor and menaced by a genocidal maniac bent on world domination. Good and evil were sharply differentiated, and American soldiers went into combat to fight a well-defined enemy with clarity of purpose.

The Vietcong, in contrast, never threatened our country or people. They were ideological adversaries, merely advocating a system of government for their tiny, impoverished nation that was different from our own. Our government's stated reason for fighting them was murky and shifting. While the South Vietnamese were our allies, they looked and talked remarkably like the northern Vietnamese we were supposed to be killing. American soldiers were fighting for an abstract political principle in a distant, steamy jungle filled with lethal traps and labyrinthine tunnels, against an enemy who was often indistinguishable from our allies. Ambiguity in a soldier's motivation for killing an adversary seems to intensify feelings of guilt; it was easier to make peace with killing a genocidal Nazi storm trooper invading France than a Vietnamese farmer whose only crime was his preference for Communism.

The difference in America's attitude toward World War II and Vietnam is reflected by the contrast between the monuments to the two wars in Washington, DC. The World War II monument is reminiscent of Roman civil architecture, with a fountain and noble pillars and bas-relief depictions of soldiers taking oaths, engaging in heroic combat, and burying the dead. There are two Vietnam memorials. The first is Maya Lin's funereal black wall representing a wound gashed into the earth with the names of the 58,209 dead inscribed on its face, while across from it stands a more conventional statue depicting three soldiers in bronze. But instead of being portrayed in

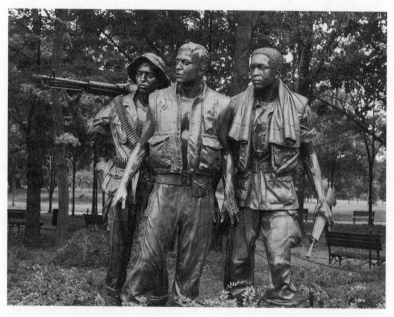

"The Three Soldiers" Vietnam Monument by Frederick Hart in Washington, DC. (Carol M. Highsmith's "America," Library of Congress Prints and Photographs Division)

a patriotic pose like the iconic raising of the American flag at Iwo Jima, the three Vietnam soldiers gaze out lifelessly in a "thousand-yard stare," a classic sign of combat trauma. (Ironically, the term "thousand-yard stare" originated in a 1944 painting of a U.S. Marine serving in the Pacific titled *The Two-Thousand Yard Stare*.) Instead of celebrating heroism and nationalism, the Vietnam War statue memorializes the terrible psychic toll on its combatants while the Wall symbolizes the psychic toll on the country.

Despite the apparent progress in the treatment of "combat exhaustion" during World War II, at the height of the Vietnam War psychological trauma was still as poorly understood as schizophrenia was during the era of "schizophrenogenic mothers." While psychoanalytically oriented treatments did seem to improve the condition of many traumatized soldiers, other soldiers seemed to get worse over time. It is astonishing, in retrospect, to consider how little was done to advance medical knowledge about psychological trauma between World War I and Vietnam, when such enormous strides were made in military medicine. In World War I, over 80 percent of combat casualties died. In the recent wars in Iraq and Afghanistan, over 80 percent of combat casualties survive as a result of the spectacular improvements in trauma surgery and medicine. PTSD, due to greater recognition but lack of scientific progress, has become the signature wound of twenty-first-century soldiers.

Rap Sessions

When traumatized Vietnam veterans returned home, they were greeted by a hostile public and an almost complete absence of medical knowledge about their condition. Abandoned and scorned, these traumatized veterans found an unlikely champion for their cause.

Chaim Shatan was a Polish-born psychoanalyst who moved to New York City in 1949 and started a private practice. Shatan was a pacifist, and in 1967 he attended an antiwar rally where he met Robert Jay Lifton, a Yale psychiatrist who shared Shatan's antiwar sentiments. The two men also discovered they shared something else in common: an interest in the psychological effects of war.

Lifton had spent years contemplating the nature of the emotional trauma endured by Hiroshima victims (eventually publishing his insightful analysis in the book *Survivors of Hiroshima*). Then, in the late '60s, he was introduced to a veteran who had been present at the My Lai Massacre, a notorious incident where American soldiers slaughtered hundreds of unarmed Vietnamese civilians. Through this veteran, Lifton became involved with a group of Vietnam veterans who regularly got together to share their experiences with one another. They called these meetings "rap sessions."

"These men were hurting and isolated," Lifton recounts. "They didn't have anybody else to talk to. The Veterans Administration was providing very little support, and civilians, including friends and family, couldn't really understand. The only people who could relate to their experiences were other vets."

Around 1970, Lifton invited his new friend Shatan to attend a rap session in New York. By the end of the meeting, Shatan was pale. These veterans had witnessed or participated in unimaginable atrocities—some had been ordered to shoot women and children and even babies—and they described these gruesome events in graphic detail. Shatan immediately realized that these rap sessions held the potential to illuminate the psychological effects of combat trauma.

"It was an opportunity to develop a new therapeutic paradigm," Lifton explains. "We didn't see the vets as a clinical population with a clinical diagnosis, at least not at the time. It was a very collegial and collaborative environment. The vets knew about the war, and the shrinks knew a little about what made people tick."

Shatan gradually appreciated that the veterans were experiencing a consistent set of psychological symptoms from their wartime experiences, and that their condition did not conform to the explanations provided by psychoanalytical theory. Shatan was trained in the Freudian doctrine, which held that combat neurosis "unmasked" negative experiences from childhood, but he recognized that these veterans were reacting to their recent wartime experiences themselves rather than anything buried in their past.

"We came to realize just how amazingly neglected the study of trauma was in psychiatry," Lifton remembers. "There was no meaningful understanding of trauma. I mean, this was a time when German biological psychiatrists were contesting their country's restitution payments to Holocaust survivors, because they claimed that there had to be a 'preexisting tendency towards illness' which was responsible for any pathogenic effects."

Working in these unstructured, egalitarian, and decidedly antiwar rap sessions, Shatan meticulously assembled a clinical picture of wartime trauma, a picture quite different from the prevailing view. On May 6, 1972, he published an article in the *New York Times* in which he publicly described his findings for the first time, and added his own appellation to the conditions previously described as soldier's heart, shell shock, battle fatigue, and combat neurosis: "Post-Vietnam Syndrome."

In the article, Shatan wrote that Post-Vietnam Syndrome manifested itself fully after a veteran returned from Asia. The soldier would experience "growing apathy, cynicism, alienation, depression, mistrust and expectation of betrayal, as well as an inability to concentrate, insomnia, nightmares, restlessness, rootlessness, and impatience with almost any job or course of study." Shatan identified a heavy moral component to veterans' suffering, including guilt, revulsion, and self-punishment. Shatan emphasized that the most poignant feature of Post-Vietnam Syndrome was a veteran's agonizing doubt about his ability to love others and to be loved.

Shatan's new clinical syndrome immediately became fodder for the polarized politics over the Vietnam War. Supporters of the war denied that combat had any psychiatric effects on soldiers at all, while opponents of the war embraced Post-Vietnam Syndrome and insisted it would cripple the military and overwhelm hospitals, leading to a national medical crisis. Hawkish psychiatrists retorted that the *DSM-II* did not even recognize combat exhaustion; the Nixon administration began harassing Shatan and Lifton as antiwar activists, and the FBI monitored their mail. Dovish psychiatrists responded by wildly exaggerating the consequences of Post-Vietnam Syndrome and the potential for violence in its victims, a conviction that soon turned into a caricature of demented danger.

A 1975 *Baltimore Sun* headline referred to returning Vietnam veterans as "Time Bombs." Four months later, the prominent *New York Times* columnist Tom Wicker told the story of a Vietnam veteran who slept with a gun under his pillow and shot his wife during a nightmare: "This is only one example of the serious but largely unnoticed problem of Post-Vietnam Syndrome."

The image of the Vietnam vet as a "trip-wire killer" was seized upon by Hollywood. In Martin Scorsese's 1976 film *Taxi Driver*, Robert De Niro is unable to distinguish between the New York present and his Vietnam past, driving him to murder. In the 1978 film *Coming Home*, Bruce Dern plays a traumatized vet, unable to readjust after returning to the States, who threatens to kill his wife (Jane Fonda) and his wife's new paramour, a paraplegic vet played by Jon Voight, before finally killing himself.

While the public came to believe that many returning veterans needed psychiatric care, most veterans found little solace in shrinks, who tried to goad their patients into finding the source of their anguish within themselves. The rap sessions, on the other hand, became a powerful source of comfort and healing. Hearing the experiences of other men who were going through the same thing helped vets to make sense of their own pain and suffering. The Veterans Administration eventually recognized the therapeutic benefits of the rap sessions and reached out to Shatan and Lifton to emulate their methods on a wider scale.

Meanwhile, Shatan and Lifton puzzled over the process by which Post-Vietnam Syndrome produced such dramatic and debilitating effects in its victims. One clue lay in its similarity to the emotional trauma in other groups of victims, such as the Hiroshima survivors documented by Lifton, as well as those who were imprisoned in Nazi concentration camps. Many Holocaust survivors aged prematurely, confused the present with the past, and suffered from depression, anxiety, and nightmares. Having learned to function in a world without morality or humanity, these survivors often found it difficult to relate to ordinary people in ordinary situations.

Shatan concluded that Post-Vietnam Syndrome, as a particular form of psychological trauma, was a legitimate mental illness—and should be formally acknowledged as such. Although the Vietnam War was raging in the late 1960s as the *DSM-II* was being assembled, no diagnosis specific to psychological trauma, let alone combat trauma, was included. As had been the case with *DSM-I*, trauma-related symptoms were classified under a broad diagnostic rubric, "adjustment reaction to adult life." Veterans who had watched children bayoneted and comrades burned alive were understandably outraged when informed that they had "a problem in adult adjustment."

When Shatan learned that the *DSM* was undergoing revision and that the Task Force was not planning to include any kind of diagnosis for trauma, he knew he had to take action. In 1975, he arranged to meet with Robert Spitzer, who he already knew professionally, at the APA annual meeting in Anaheim, California, and lobbied vehemently for the inclusion of Post-Vietnam Syndrome in *DSM-III.* Initially, Spitzer was skeptical of Shatan's proposed syndrome. But Shatan persevered, sending Spitzer reams of information describing the symptoms, including Lifton's work on Hiroshima victims—the kind of diagnostic data that was always sure to get Spitzer's attention. Spitzer eventually relented and in 1977 agreed to create a Committee on Reactive Disorders and assigned one of his Task Force members, Nancy Andreasen, the job of formally vetting Shatan's proposal.

Andreasen was a smart and tough-minded psychiatrist who had worked in the Burn Unit of New York Hospital–Cornell Medical Center as a medical student, an experience that would shape her attitude toward Post-Vietnam Syndrome. "Bob Spitzer asked me to deal with Shatan's Syndrome," Andreasen explained, "but he did not know that I was already an expert on the topic of stress-induced neuropsychiatric disorders. I began my psychiatry career by studying the physical and mental consequences of one of the most horrible stresses that human beings can experience: severe burn injuries."

Gradually, Andreasen came to agree with Shatan's conclusions: that a consistent syndrome of symptoms could develop from any traumatic event, whether losing your home in a fire, getting mugged in a park, or being in a firefight during combat. Since she had previously classified the psychology of burn victims as "stress-induced disorders," Andreasen christened her broadened conceptualization of Post-Vietnam Syndrome as "Post-Traumatic Stress Disorder" and proposed the following summary: "The essential feature is the development of characteristic symptoms following a psychologically traumatic event that is generally outside the range of usual human experience."

Despite the meager scientific evidence available on the disorder beyond Shatan and Lifton's observations from the veteran rap groups, the Task Force accepted Andreasen's proposal with little opposition. Spitzer later acknowledged to me that if Shatan had not pressed his case for Post-Vietnam Syndrome, most likely it would never have ended up in the *DSM-III*.

Since then, traumatized veterans have had a much easier time getting the medical attention they need, since both the military and psychiatry finally acknowledged that they were suffering from a genuine medical condition.

But while the *DSM-III* bestowed legitimacy on the suffering of soldiers traumatized in war—as well as the suffering of victims of rape, assault, torture, burns, bombings, natural disasters, and financial catastrophe—when the *Manual* was published in 1980, psychiatrists still knew precious little about the pathological basis of PTSD and what might be going on in the brains of its victims.

A Fear of Fireworks

The Kronskys were barely forty and enjoyed a happy marriage. He was a successful accountant. She translated foreign-language books into English. But the focus of their life was their two rambunctious children: twelve-year-old Ellie and ten-year-old Edmund. One evening, Mr. and Mrs. Kronsky and Edmund attended a holiday dinner at a friend's home. (Ellie spent the night at a classmate's birthday sleepover party.) After a festive dinner, the Kronskys climbed into their car and headed home on familiar roads. Edmund yawned and expressed disappointment that he had missed the Knicks game, though Mr. Kronsky assured him that they had taped it and Edmund could watch it tomorrow. And then, without warning, their lives changed forever.

As the Kronskys passed through an intersection, a speeding SUV hurtled through a red light and slammed into the rear of their car on the passenger side. Edmund was sitting in the back seat with his seatbelt unbuckled. The rear doors crumpled and wrenched open, and Edmund was thrown out of the car into the middle of the intersection. A large pickup truck was bearing down on the intersection from the opposite direction.

The driver of the pickup had no time to swerve, and Mr. and Mrs. Kronsky watched in horror as the vehicle rolled over Edmund's body. Despite the rapid arrival of an EMS team, the boy could not be saved.

For the next two years the Kronksys grieved together, avoiding friends and family. Then, ever so gradually, Mrs. Kronsky started to recover. First, she began translating books again. Then she reached out to their old friends, and eventually started going to the movies with them and sharing a meal afterwards. Though she could never fully let go of the tragedy of losing her son, by the end of the third year she had resumed most of the routines of her former life.

For Mr. Kronsky, it was a different story. Two years after the accident, he was still visiting his son's grave almost every day. He had no interest in any social activities, even after his wife began seeing their friends again. He was always irritable and distracted. Sloppy mistakes began to creep into his accounting work. Loyal clients went to other firms. While he had previously managed his family's finances with obsessive fastidiousness, he now ignored them almost completely. His entire universe consisted of a single memory repeated over and over, day after day: the pickup trampling his small, frightened son.

As Mrs. Kronsky continued to recover, Mr. Kronsky only grew worse. He drank heavily and provoked explosive arguments with his wife, which is what prompted them to see me. After our first session, it was clear that Mr. Kronsky was suffering from PTSD and a complicated grief reaction. I worked with them for a few months and helped wean Mr. Kronsky off alcohol. Antidepressant medication helped mitigate some of his more severe mood swings and his outbursts of rage, and eventually the marital discord diminished—or at least the number of fights decreased. But other problems persisted.

Despite my best efforts, Mr. Kronsky was unable to function effectively at work and failed to resume any of his former social and recreational activities. Most of the time he sat at home watching television, at least until some program triggered a memory of his son's death and he swiftly flicked it off. With his business collapsing, his wife became the breadwinner; this became a source of increasing tension, since he resented that she was the one providing for their family. Meanwhile, she grew increasingly frustrated with her husband's unwillingness to even *try* to do anything outside of their home.

Finally, Mrs. Kronsky decided she could no longer live with a disabled husband who refused to try to move on. She believed their home was an unhealthy environment for her daughter, who came home from school each day to inevitably find an angry father sulking around the house or curled up on the sofa—a father who treated Ellie as if she was dead, too. Finally, Mrs. Kronsky moved out with her daughter and filed for divorce. She continued her career, saw her daughter go off to college, and eventually remarried. Mr. Kronsky's life had a much different outcome.

Unable to overcome the horrific event that cost him his son, he returned to his abuse of alcohol and eventually cut me off, too. When I last interacted with him, he remained trapped in a bleak, isolated existence, avoiding all contact with other people, including those who wished to help him.

Why did Mr. Kronsky develop post-traumatic stress disorder and not Mrs. Kronsky, even though they both experienced the same trauma? When the *DSM-III* Task Force voted to authorize PTSD, there was no knowledge about how trauma produced its immediate and enduring effects and no understanding of how to alleviate its consequences. If a soldier is hit in the head by flying shrapnel, we know what to do: stop the bleeding, clean and bandage the wound, get X-rays to assess any internal damage. PTSD, in contrast, was a complete mystery. If this is a serious mental illness with a clear-cut cause, shouldn't we be able to figure out *something* about how it works?

Once PTSD was legitimized by its inclusion in *DSM-III*, funding for research on the disorder started pouring in. However, it required the "brain revolution" in psychiatry—the new brain-imaging techniques in the 1980s and the increasing number of psychiatric neuroscientists inspired by Eric Kandel—before researchers could make headway and begin to understand the intricate neural architecture of the brain that underlies PTSD. Gradually, in the 2000s, new brain-focused research revealed the pathological process that is believed to cause the condition.

This process involves three key brain structures: the amygdala, the prefrontal cortex, and the hippocampus. These three structures form a neural circuit that is essential for learning from emotionally arousing experiences, but if an experience is *too* extreme, the circuit can turn against itself. For example, imagine you are visiting Yellowstone National Park. You stop your car to take a stroll in the woods. Suddenly, you spot a huge bear not far away. You immediately feel a rush of fear because your amygdala, a part of your primordial emotional system, has sounded the alarm for danger and signaled for you to flee. What should you do?

Your brain has evolved to help you to survive and enable you to make the best split-second decisions in life-threatening situations. Though your amygdala is screaming at you to run for your life, the most beneficial course of action is to hold your amygdala-stoked emotions in check while you analyze the situation and choose the best option. Perhaps you are more likely to survive if you stand still so that the bear won't notice you, perhaps you should yell and make loud noises to frighten it or pick up a large stick to defend yourself, or perhaps the smartest option is to pull out your cell phone and call the park rangers. But you will only be able to make a decision if you consciously overcome your emotional urges, a process that neuroscientists call *cognitive control*. Your decision making and cognitive control are handled by the newest and most highly evolved part of your brain, the prefrontal cortex. The more experienced and mature we are, the more likely our prefrontal cortex will be able to exert cognitive control and override our amygdala's insistent impulse to flee.

But let's say that you are so scared that your prefrontal cortex can't counteract your fear. Your amygdala wins out and you start racing for your car as fast as your feet will carry you. The bear spots you and, with a loud growl, gives chase. Fortunately, you outrace the bear, making it to your car and slamming the door just as the bear lunges at you. You've survived. Your brain is designed to learn from this valuable life-preserving experience. Your hippocampus now forms a long-term memory of the bear and your decision to flee, a memory that is emotionally saturated with the amygdala's fear.

The primary reason for the existence of your amygdala–prefrontal cortex–hippocampus system is to enable you to learn from your experiences and improve your ability to react to similar circumstances in the future. The next time you encounter a bear (or a wolf, or a boar, or a cougar) in the woods (or a jungle, or a field), your stored memory will be triggered by the event's similarity to your original bear encounter and the memory will automatically guide you to react swiftly: *Holy cow, another bear? I survived by running last time, so I better run again!*

But what if your original experience fleeing the bear was so traumatic and terrifying that your amygdala lit up like Times Square? Maybe the bear caught up to you before you reached the car and managed to claw your back before you hopped inside. Then it's possible that your amygdala was firing so wildly it forged a traumatic memory in your hippocampus with searing emotional intensity. Since the stored memory is so powerful, when it is triggered it overwhelms your prefrontal cortex and prevents you from exercising cognitive control. Moreover, in the future the memory might be triggered by stimuli that only vaguely resemble the original event, such that the next time you saw any furry animal—even your neighbor's poodle—the sight might trigger your original memory, causing your amygdala to instinctively react as if you are again being threatened by a deadly bear—*Holy cow, I better run again!*

In other words, individuals afflicted with PTSD cannot separate the details of a new experience from the emotional charge of a past trauma and cannot prevent their amygdala-hippocampus circuit from reliving the mental intensity of the original event. This is what happened to Adrianne Haslet.

On a bright, sunny Patriots' Day in 2013, Adrianne Haslet stood near the finish line of the Boston marathon, a few yards away from an explosive-laden stainless-steel pressure cooker stuffed in an abandoned backpack. When it exploded, her foot was blown off. The experience would be horrific for anyone—but it was especially traumatic for Adrianne, a dancer who had devoted her life to the nimble use of her feet. Her amygdala maxed out, sending a blistering emotional signal to her hippocampus, which stored a hyperpotent memory of the explosion and its grisly aftermath.

A few months later, after her discharge from Mass General Hospital, Adrianne was back in her Boston apartment when she was suddenly startled by another series of loud explosions—the city's Fourth of July fireworks display. The sounds of the holiday pyrotechnics ripped through her brain and instantly activated her memory of the marathon explosion, forcing her to relive the same feelings of terror she felt while lying on the blood-drenched sidewalk on Boylston Street. Frantic, she called 911 and begged the helpless dispatcher to halt the fireworks.

Most of us have experienced a milder, nonpathological form of this neural phenomenon during events that are dramatic and unexpected but not quite horrifying. Many people can remember where they were when they heard that President Reagan was shot or learned about the Challenger space shuttle explosion or watched the September 11 attacks unfold. These are sometimes called "flashbulb memories," and they are the benign non–emotion laden equivalent of the searing, mind-bending memories that PTSD victims can't get out of their heads.

Using knowledge of the neural mechanism of trauma, recent research has shown that if a person takes a memory-disrupting drug shortly after a traumatic experience—even hours later—PTSD can be drastically reduced, since the hippocampus is prevented from fully consolidating what would become a traumatic memory. (This research was grounded in Eric Kandel's work demonstrating how short-term memories are encoded into long-term memory.) Research also points to genetic variability in our susceptibility to PTSD. Specific genes involved with the brain mechanisms that control arousal, anxiety, and vigilance seem to be correlated with whether or not a person develops PTSD symptoms. While every person has a breaking point and is capable of developing PTSD if stressed long or hard enough, each person's breaking point is different.

The dynamics of the amygdala–prefrontal cortex–hippo-campus circuit may help explain why I developed my own PTSD-like symptoms after I dropped the air conditioner but not after my home invasion, and why Mr. Kronsky developed intractable symptoms following the death of his son, while Mrs. Kronsky recovered. The crucial factor was cognitive control.

When I was being robbed, my prefrontal cortex enabled me to keep my cool and gave me the sense (however illusory it may have been) that I was in control through the belief that if I made the decision to obey my attackers I would survive unharmed. Since I escaped without serious injury or signifi-cant loss, my hippocampus committed to memory an experi-ence that was tempered by my sense of cognitive control. In contrast, once the air conditioner slipped from my fingers, there was absolutely nothing I could do other than shout impo-tently as it plummeted toward the sidewalk. There was no con-trol, real or illusory, to mitigate my amygdala's blaring alarm. Thus my hippocampus stored a memory of the experience that was as vivid as a sports arena Jumbotron.

The situation was different with Mr. Kronsky. The fact that he was driving the car would seem to have given him some sense of cognitive as well as physical control over the situation. However, in reality, Kronsky had little influence over the acci-dent's circumstances in which he was both a passive victim and an observer. Consequently, his hippocampus likely stored a memory that combined the emotional intensity of Edmund's grisly demise with the guilt-ridden awareness of his role behind the wheel. In this case, his sense of cognitive control became a mental prison, plaguing him with endless "what ifs": "what if I had not wanted to leave the party early?" "what if I had taken a different route home?" "what if I had driven more slowly through the intersection?"

Since I survived my home invasion unscathed, my own

sense of cognitive control helped mitigate the emotional intensity of the experience. But if the two thugs who broke into my apartment had ended up shooting me or stealing my grandfather's watch, then the same decision to stay calm might have instead thrust me into my own never-ending labyrinth of self-recrimination. Such is the relationship between the brain and our experiences. That which can teach us can also wound us.

Chapter 9

The Triumph of Pluralism: The *DSM-5*

Psychiatry is neurology without physical signs, and calls for diagnostic virtuosity of the highest order.

— HENRY GEORGE MILLER, BRITISH JOURNAL OF
HOSPITAL MEDICINE, 1970

I identify humility rather than hubris as the proper basis of scientific maturity. The ideal is not truth or certainty, but a continual and pluralistic pursuit of knowledge.

— HASOK CHANG

Diagnosis in the Digital Age

The fourth edition of the Bible of Psychiatry was published in 1994. It contained 297 disorders (up from 265) and followed the same framework that Spitzer had laid out in the *DSM-III*. While the publication of the *DSM-III* had been marked by tumult and controversy, the release of the *DSM-IV* was as routine and uneventful as the opening of a Starbucks. Most mental health professionals hardly noticed the process of its construction; they simply began using it when it was released.

The fifth edition, however, was a different story. In 2006, the APA officially authorized the appointment of a new Task Force to develop the *DSM-5*. Much had changed in the world of medicine and psychiatry since the paradigm-shattering *DSM-III* was released in 1980. President George H. W. Bush had proclaimed the 1990s the Decade of the Brain, and neuroscience had burgeoned into one of the most important and dynamic disciplines in the life sciences. Imaging and genetics thoroughly permeated the medical field. There was an abundance of new drugs, new psychotherapy techniques, and new medical devices and technologies.

At the same time, the power and functionality of computers had increased drastically, and the Internet had become a pervasive social force.

In recognition of the new digital era into which the fifth edition would be born, the *Manual*'s abbreviation was changed to *DSM-5* instead of *DSM-V*. By replacing the Roman numeral with a number, the APA suggested that the *DSM* would now be a "living document" and revised iteratively like computer software, and promised the possible release of a *DSM-5.1* and *5.2*.

In 2006, APA president Steve Sharfstein appointed David Kupfer as chair of the Task Force and Darrel Regier as vice chair. Kupfer was the chair of the psychiatry department at the University of Pittsburgh and a world-renowned expert in depression and bipolar disorder. Regier was a psychiatrist and epidemiologist who had cut his teeth on the landmark Epidemiologic Catchment Study, a 1980s NIMH project that measured the rates of mental disorders in the American population.

Kupfer and Regier assembled their team, which went to work in 2007. Like previous *DSM* Task Forces, they conducted extensive literature reviews, analyzed data, and solicited feedback from colleagues and professionals to help them formulate revisions to the existing diagnoses. But unlike previous Task Forces, muffled complaints could soon be heard: There wasn't a consistent set of procedures for changing diagnoses; there wasn't a clear plan for assembling the diagnoses into a new edition. In addition, interested parties, both within and outside the profession, observed that the process of reviewing and revising the *DSM* was being orchestrated behind closed doors. Hearing rumblings of discontent, a new generation of antipsychiatry activists, including Robert Whittaker,

Gary Greenberg, Peter Breggin, and a reinvigorated Church of Scientology, began to take swipes at the project.

This wasn't the '70s, when criticism of the *DSM-III* unfolded almost entirely within the insular world of the mental health profession, with opponents jousting through journal commentaries, typewritten letters, and private meetings. This was the twenty-first century, the age of the Internet and social media. Even nonprofessionals were now empowered to communicate their grievances through blogs, online newsletters, activist websites, Facebook posts, and eventually Twitter. Capturing the spirit of much of the early criticism of the *DSM-5*, Gary Greenberg, a psychotherapist and writer of antipsychiatry screeds, declared in a *New York Times* interview, "No one puts much stock in the actual content of the *DSM*, and even those who defend it acknowledge that its primary virtue is that there isn't anything else to use."

The familiar antipsychiatry critics were next joined by voices from stakeholder groups who wanted to know how the *DSM* process would affect their constituencies. Patient advocacy organizations such as the National Alliance for the Mentally Ill, Autism Speaks, the Depression and Bipolar Support Alliance, and the American Foundation for Suicide Prevention also began to complain online that their constituents were being kept in the dark about the formative *DSM-5* process. Soon, there were myriad blogs and online discussions castigating the opaqueness of the *DSM-5*'s development. By failing to respond to this flurry of online salvos, the APA and the *DSM-5* Task Force gave the impression that those in charge were not taking the complaints seriously — or were simply out of touch.

In truth, the APA really was caught flat-footed by the mounting online criticism. Not only were they ill-equipped to use the Internet to respond in an organized or effective fashion, they were completely taken by surprise by the level of public interest. After all, during the development of the

DSM-IV there had been precious little controversy among medical professionals, while public discussion had been virtually nonexistent. But now there were hundreds of voices calling for the *DSM* leaders to pull back the curtain and explain exactly how the next generation of psychiatric diagnoses were being created.

Despite the outcry, it was possible for the Task Force chairs and APA leadership to dismiss the complaints as the usual carping and hyperbole coming from rabid antipsychiatry critics and special interest groups. After all, many of the objections leveled against the *DSM-5* process weren't all that different from the griping during the construction of the *DSM-III* and (to a lesser extent) the *DSM-IV*; they were simply amplified by the digital megaphone of the Internet. With so many individuals and entities holding a stake in the Bible of Psychiatry, any revision was sure to ruffle feathers and provoke kvetching. The APA hoped that they might be able to weather the online storm without getting wet... until a most unexpected pair of critics spoke out with the force of a hurricane.

These psychiatrists stunned the *DSM-5* leadership with a series of excoriating online missives that would eventually force the APA to alter the course of the book's development. The first psychiatrist was the chair of the *DSM-IV*, Allen Frances. The second was the legendary architect of the modern Kraepelinian *DSM*, Robert Spitzer himself.

Critics Emeritus

In April of 2007, one year after work on the *DSM-5* officially began and six years before it was scheduled for publication, Robert Spitzer sent a two-line message to *DSM-5* vice chair Darrel Regier. Would it be possible for Regier to forward to him a copy of the minutes of the Task Force's initial meetings?

After completing the *DSM-III*, Spitzer's role in the *DSM* process had become diminished. He had lobbied hard to lead the *DSM-IV* but was passed over in favor of Allen Frances, then a professor of psychiatry at Cornell Medical College. Nevertheless, Frances had treated Spitzer respectfully, appointing him to the *DSM-IV* Task Force as a "special advisor" and including him in all meetings. But as the *DSM-5* was gearing up, Spitzer was excluded from any involvement (as was Allen Frances). Just as Spitzer had done thirty years ago, it appeared that Kupfer and Regier wanted to make a clean break with the past and create something new. In order to achieve their ambitious goal, they felt they needed to keep any previous *DSM* leadership at arm's length.

Regier responded to Spitzer by saying that minutes would be made available to the public after the conflict of interest process had been finalized and the Task Force fully approved. Spitzer wrote to Regier again a few months later but received no response. In February of 2008, almost a year after his initial request, Spitzer finally got a definitive answer to his inquiry: Due to "unprecedented" circumstances, including the need for "confidentiality in the development process," Regier and Kupfer had decided that the minutes would only be made available to the board of trustees and the members of the Task Force itself.

This wasn't merely a personal snub directed at the architect of the modern *DSM* but a severe departure from Spitzer's policy of transparency and engagement, a policy he had maintained even when confronted with pitched resistance to the *DSM-III*. Allen Frances had continued Spitzer's policy of openness during the development of the *DSM-IV*. Concerned that Regier and Kupfer's decision to close off all proceedings from public view would endanger both the legitimacy and quality of the *DSM-5*, Spitzer did something that no one expected: He took his concerns to the Web.

"The June 6th issue of *Psychiatric News* brought the good news that the *DSM-5* process will be complex but transparent," Spitzer wrote in an open letter to the editor of APA's online news service. "I found out how transparent and open when Regier informed me that he would not send me the minutes of the *DSM-5* Task Force meetings because it was important to 'maintain *DSM-5* confidentiality.'" Galvanized into action, Spitzer began an unrelenting online campaign against the "secrecy" of the *DSM-5* process and urging full transparency. "Anything less," he wrote in 2008, "is an invitation to critics of psychiatric diagnosis to raise questions about the scientific credibility of the *DSM-5*." He also criticized the use of the "confidentiality agreements" that all Task Force and work group members had been required to sign, prohibiting them from discussing the *DSM-5* outside of the Task Force and work groups.

Apparently Kupfer and Regier believed they could more effectively control the creation of a new *DSM* by shielding its Task Force and work groups from public scrutiny while they labored at the complex and potentially contentious job of improving psychiatric diagnoses. Spitzer himself had maintained an iron grip on the development of the *DSM-III*, but he had balanced his obsessive governance with an open and responsive operation, sending out a continuous stream of updates and reports. Even when he faced overt hostility in the latter stages of the *DSM-III*'s development, he famously responded to every letter, article, and phone call that inquired about the *DSM-III*, no matter how critical.

Spitzer wasn't the only one vexed by the secrecy of the *DSM-5* process. Allen Frances shared his former mentor's skepticism. Frances had trained at Columbia under Spitzer and was one of the youngest members of the *DSM-III* Task Force before becoming chair of the *DSM-IV*; the general opinion among mental health professionals was that Frances had done a respectable job as steward of psychiatry's most important book. Frances reached out to Spitzer, and in 2009, the two psychiatric luminaries posted a joint letter to the APA Board of Trustees warning that the *DSM-5* was headed for "disastrous unintended consequences" because of a "rigid fortress mentality" by which its leadership "sealed itself off from advice and criticism." They urged the APA to scrap all confidentiality agreements, increase transparency, and appoint an oversight committee to monitor the *DSM-5* process.

A firestorm erupted. At issue was the question of how to define mental illnesses in the digital age. Not only did far more empirical data and clinical knowledge exist than ever before, but there were myriad powerful stakeholders—including commercial, governmental, medical, and educational institutions, as well as patient advocacy groups—who would be significantly affected by any changes in the *DSM*. Would the public's interests be served by allowing experts to work on revisions behind a protective veil? Or was it better to allow the debates over diagnoses (which would inevitably be heated and contentious) to play out before the public eye—which now consisted of a whole wired world of bloggers, tweeters, and Facebook users?

Both defenders and detractors of the APA weighed in. The *Psychiatric Times*, an online magazine independent from the APA, published retorts on a regular basis. Daniel Carlat, a psychiatrist affiliated with Tufts University School of Medicine, described the ensuing conflict on his blog: "What began as a group of top scientists reviewing the research literature has degenerated into a dispute that puts the Hatfield-McCoy feud to shame." The media, animated by the spectacle of the most prominent practitioners in the field warring with one another with the same rancor as the Republicans and Democrats in Congress, added fuel to the fire. Cable news shows invited talking heads to debate the merits of the *DSM*, and psychiatry in general. Prominent commentators from David Brooks to Bill

O'Reilly weighed in. "The problem is that the behavioral sciences like psychiatry are not really sciences; they are semisciences," wrote Brooks in an op-ed piece in the *New York Times*.

From 2008 until the launch of the *DSM-5* in 2013, almost three thousand articles about the *DSM-5* appeared in newspapers and major online news outlets. It got to the point where minor milestones in the development of the *DSM-5* drove the news, while any news event related to mental illness was immediately referred back to the controversial status of the *Manual*. In 2011, for instance, there was an explosion in news coverage of the *DSM-5* when Congresswoman Gabrielle Giffords was shot at an Arizona shopping mall by a psychotic young man. Another *DSM-5* media frenzy followed the horrific 2012 school shooting in Newtown, Connecticut, once reports suggested that the perpetrator, Adam Lanza, had some form of autism. Much of the coverage suggested that psychiatry was not doing a good job of figuring out how to diagnose or treat mental illness.

The APA hadn't experienced this kind of public pressure since the early 1970s, when the Rosenhan study, the homosexuality controversy, and the antipsychiatry movement compelled the APA to move away from psychoanalysis and endorse a radically new paradigm for psychiatric diagnosis. But what would the APA do this time?

The APA Responds

Throughout the development process, Kupfer and Regier had repeatedly assured the APA Board in their regular reports that—despite all the internal grumbling and external noise—everything was going well with the *DSM-5*. But when Spitzer and Frances joined the online fray and the rumors about poor leadership drifting out of the Task Force and work groups failed to abate, the board began to wonder if there might be a fire behind all that smoke. Were there serious problems with the *DSM-5* development process that Kupfer and Regier were not admitting—or even worse, problems they were not aware of?

To find out, the APA Board of Trustees appointed an oversight committee in 2009. The new committee would examine the *DSM-5* process and inform the board whether there were in fact problems requiring the board's intervention. Carolyn Robinowitz, former dean of the Georgetown University School of Medicine and a previous APA president, was appointed chair of the committee. I was also appointed to the committee.

We attended the *DSM* Task Force meetings, where we were updated by the *DSM-5* chair and vice chair, and then met separately with task force members without Kupfer or Regier present. It quickly became apparent that the situation was as bad as the rumors had suggested. The *DSM-III* team had been unified in their vision of a new *Manual* and had complete confidence in Robert Spitzer's leadership. With the *DSM-5*, many team members were openly critical of both the process and its leaders.

Regier and his staff seemed disorganized and uncertain, while Kupfer was remote and disengaged, delegating operational responsibility to Regier. This was a very different management style from the obsessive hands-on involvement of Spitzer, later emulated by Frances. Robinowitz reported back to the APA Board the sobering conclusions of the oversight committee: "There is a serious problem with the *DSM*, and we've got to fix it."

The board of trustees took Robinowitz's comments to heart but was unsure what to do. To change horses in midstream when the process was being publicly questioned might lend credence to the criticism and undermine the credibility of the *DSM*. Instead, the board fashioned a workaround by establishing two ad hoc review committees: one to review the scientific evidence justifying any proposed change, and another to review the clinical and public health implications of any change. While adding new committees is hardly an ideal solution to a management problem, it did serve to deflect much of the criticism coming from within the psychiatry profession itself.

Meanwhile, the Internet was still teeming with accusations. One of the most prominent was the claim that the *DSM-5* was pathologizing normal behavior. Ironically, the pathologization of the ordinary had been one of Robert Spitzer's most pointed criticisms of the psychoanalysts, who quite explicitly talked about the psychopathology of everyday life and argued that everyone was a little mentally ill. One of the great contributions of Spitzer and the *DSM-III* was to draw a bright, clear line between the mentally ill and the mentally well, and even within the chaos of the *DSM-5* that division was being adhered to.

Most of the invective about pathologizing normal behavior was provoked by diagnoses that sounded trivial or sexist to casual observers, such as hoarding disorder, binge eating disorder, and premenstrual dysphoric disorder. Yet the case for designating each of these conditions a disorder was supported by data or extensive clinical experience. Take hoarding disorder, one of the new entries in the *DSM-5*. This condition is associated with the compulsive inability to throw things away, to the point where detritus obstructs one's living environment and substantially reduces the quality of one's life. Though we all know pack rats who are reluctant to throw away old items, individuals suffering from hoarding disorder often accumulate so much *stuff* that the looming heaps of debris can present a serious health hazard.

I once treated an affluent middle-aged woman who lived in a spacious apartment on the Upper East Side of Manhattan but could barely open the door to get into or out of her apartment because of the wobbly towers of accumulated newspapers, pet magazines, unopened purchases from cable shopping networks, and accouterments for her nine cats. Finally she was threatened with eviction when neighbors complained of the foul odors and vermin emanating from her unit. Her family hospitalized her, and she was treated for the first time in her life for her hoarding disorder. Three weeks later, she was discharged and returned home to a pristine apartment that her family had cleaned out. She now takes clomipramine (a tricyclic antidepressant often used to treat obsessive-compulsive disorder) and receives cognitive-behavioral therapy to help her manage her impulses. So far, she lives a much happier life in her clean and roomy apartment, with no complaints from her neighbors or family.

As someone intimately involved with the *DSM-5* development process, I can tell you that there is no institutional interest in expanding the scope of psychiatry by inventing more disorders or making it easier to qualify for a diagnosis. We have more patients than we can possibly handle within our current mental health care system, and we already face enough challenges trying to get insurance companies to reimburse us for treating diagnoses that have been established for decades. Perhaps the strongest piece of evidence that psychiatry is not trying to pathologize ordinary behaviors can be found in the changing number of diagnoses: the *DSM-IV* had 297. The *DSM-5* reduced it to 265.

When I became president-elect of the APA in the spring of 2012, I inherited the responsibility for the *DSM-5*. It would be completed and published during my term, and its success—or failure—would play out on my watch. I was somewhat consoled by the fact that the ad hoc committees established by my predecessors had been effective and had substantially improved the *DSM* development process. The internal grumbling had ceased, a clear and rigorous process for creating or changing disorders was established, and most important, each tentative set of diagnostic criteria was accumulating more evidence and undergoing more deliberation than during any previous *DSM*.

In the final six months before the *DSM-5* was to be presented to the APA Assembly for a vote, APA president Dilip Jeste and I set up a systematic "Summit" process to conduct a final review and approve or reject every proposed disorder. The final set of approved diagnoses would then be presented en masse to the APA Assembly, just as occurred with Spitzer's *DSM-III* thirty years earlier. Representatives of the Task Force, work groups, and committees all participated, and every one of us knew exactly what was at stake: the credibility of psychiatry in the twenty-first century, and the welfare of every patient whose life would be affected by the decisions we made.

During the Summit review process, we always sought consensus. If there was not clear scientific evidence or a compelling clinical rationale supporting a new diagnosis or a revision to an existing diagnosis, then the version in the *DSM-IV* was left unchanged. The majority of the disorders were approved without controversy, though there was heated debate over personality disorders—a perennial source of contention among psychiatrists with roots in Freud's earliest psychoanalytical theories. There were also disagreements about whether to include a new diagnosis for children called "disruptive mood dysregulation disorder"; whether someone could be diagnosed with depression while still grieving the death of a loved one; and whether the criteria for schizophrenia should be modified. These three changes were eventually approved, though the newly proposed configuration of personality disorders was not.

Finally November 10, 2012, arrived—the day of the *DSM-5* vote. The APA Assembly convened in the JW Marriott in Washington, DC, exactly two blocks from the White House, less than a week after Barack Obama had won the right to reside there for another four years. After all of the thunderous controversy over the *DSM-5* online and in the media, when the final vote to approve it came, it was downright anticlimactic. There was very little discussion on the floor of the ballroom, and the vote itself was quick and unanimous, a far cry from the frenzied activities and last-ditch efforts to rework the *DSM-III*.

The *DSM-5* was published on May 19, 2013, concluding the longest period of development of any *DSM* (seven years) and the longest period between *DSM* editions (nineteen years). But this delay was not so much due to the controversy and unwieldy process as it was a reflection of the unprecedented scope of work that went into the *DSM-5*'s development. The new edition of the Bible of Psychiatry incorporated more data, evidence, and discussion than the previous four editions combined: 163 experts, including psychiatrists, psychologists, sociologists, nurses, and consumer advocates, devoted more than one hundred thousand hours of work, reviewed tens of thousands of papers, and obtained input on diagnostic criteria from hundreds of active clinicians. Except for the chair and vice chair, none of these contributors received any payment for their efforts.

Despite all the drama, fear, and ambition that played out during the creation of the *DSM-5*, the final product ultimately proved to be a rather modest revision of the *DSM-IV*. It retained most of the elements that Spitzer introduced in his transformative edition, including his basic definition of mental illness as a consistent and enduring pattern of symptoms that causes subjective distress or impairment of functioning.

After its launch, Jeste wrote, "the successful publication of the diagnostic manual—on a tight deadline and in the face of massive public scrutiny—is an unqualified victory for psychiatry. In May of 2012 it looked like it would be a difficult task, and there were articles appearing in the press, mostly critical. We responded to the criticism in a very constructive way, without bashing the critics. If it had not gone well, it could have been a black eye, not just for APA, but the profession of psychiatry. This has to be the most reviewed diagnostic system in the history of medicine. I think we should all take pride in this remarkable achievement."

You can count me among those who take pride in the result. But for others, the final product was a severe disappointment. Just as the *DSM-5* was being launched, the director of the National Institute of Mental Health posted a highly critical blog that caused the greatest *DSM* media uproar of them all. While Tom Insel's condemnation of the digital-age *DSM* appeared to threaten psychiatry's integrity yet again, his challenge provided an opportunity to demonstrate the true strength and resilience of contemporary psychiatry.

Toward a Pluralistic Psychiatry

In his April 29, 2013, blog, the top government psychiatrist and director of the world's largest funder of psychiatric research declared, "Patients with mental disorders deserve better than the *DSM-5*. That is why NIMH will be re-orienting its research away from *DSM* categories." Tom Insel's broadside immediately went viral, and the media reported his declaration as an official rejection of the *DSM* by the NIMH. Insel seemed to be announcing to the world that psychiatry's diagnoses were not scientifically sound. In place of the *DSM-5*, Insel advocated the creation of a new diagnostic system based upon genetics, neurobiology, brain circuits, and biomarkers.

Insel was expressing the perpetual dream of biological psychiatry to establish neural definitions of psychopathology, as first articulated by Wilhelm Griesinger and his German cohorts a century and a half ago. As we've observed over psychiatry's two centuries of history, however, most attempts at providing a biological accounting of mental illness have been stymied. Griesinger himself failed, Kraepelin turned to symptoms and illness course in frustration, Freud appreciated the futility and developed psychoanalysis, Egas Moniz's lobotomy-justifying theory of functional fixations failed, John Cade's toxin theory

of mania failed, the mauve and pink spots of the chromatography psychiatrists failed. The only undisputed biological
explanations of the origins of a mental illness are for General
Paresis of the Insane (caused by the syphilis bacteria), pellagra
(a form of dementia caused by vitamin B-12 deficiency), and
more recently Alzheimer and other forms of dementia and
drug-induced psychoses. We have a reasonable understanding
of how addiction and post-traumatic stress disorder develop in
the brain, though we still have much to learn. While biological
psychiatry has uncovered tantalizing clues, if we survey the
entire history of psychiatry, we find that biological theories of
mental illness have tended to fare no better or worse than
psychodynamic theories, with neither school of thought yet
providing a convincing accounting of the precise origins of
schizophrenia, depression, or anxiety and bipolar disorders. If
we've learned anything from the repeated pendulum swings
back and forth between brain and mind, it's that any narrow
perspective on mental illness usually proves to be inadequate
to account for the complexity that is mental illness.

Ironically, sixty years before NIMH director Tom Insel
blogged about the need to embrace a purely biological psychiatry, the first director of the NIMH, Robert Felix, denounced
biological psychiatry and declared that NIMH would not fund
any biological research (a promise he regrettably made good
on). Instead, Felix urged psychiatrists to focus on social pathologies like poverty, racism, and family strife. Later, as psychiatry's pendulum began to swing back toward the brain in the
early 1980s, propelled by advances in imaging, genetics, and
neuroscience, the chair of psychiatry at Yale, Morton Reiser,
remarked, "We are going from a brainless psychiatry to a mind-
less psychiatry."

Robert Spitzer's genius was to remain agnostic on the question of whether the biological or psychodynamic camp had
more to offer, and he created a diagnostic framework that could

incorporate research from both perspectives—or neither. The reason that genetics, neurobiology, brain circuits, and biomarkers are absent from *DSM-5* diagnoses is that there was not yet enough evidence to support their inclusion, and not because of some kind of oversight, theoretical bias, or deliberate rejection of biological psychiatry. Rather, it was a reflection of a responsible and mature view of mental illness embodied in the *DSM*'s dispassionate attitude toward psychiatric theorizing. Ultimately it was the empirical data that mattered, as recalcitrant or uninnovative or same-old as that data might be.

The wild conceptual gyrations throughout the history of psychiatry underscore the value of Spitzer's open-minded agnosticism, since psychiatry has always fared best when it managed to avoid both extremes of reductionist neurobiology and pure mentalism, instead pursuing a path of moderation that is receptive to findings from all empirically based sources. Though it's still possible to find individual psychiatrists today who adhere exclusively to a psychodynamic, biological, or sociological perspective, the field of psychiatry as a whole has come to realize that the best way to understand and treat mental illness is by simultaneously addressing the mind *and* the brain.

Today, psychiatrists are trained to evaluate their patients using the latest techniques of neuroscience *and* the most cogent psychodynamic principles of mental function. They use brain-imaging technology *and* carefully listen to patients' accounts of their experiences, emotions, and desires. Ken Kendler, professor of psychiatry and human genetics at Virginia Commonwealth University and one of the most cited psychiatric researchers alive, has characterized this unified, open-minded approach to mental illness as "pluralistic psychiatry."

In an insightful 2014 paper, Kendler cautions the newly dominant psychiatric neuroscientists against the "fervent monism" that characterized the psychoanalysts of the 1940s and '50s and the social psychiatrists of the 1960s and '70s, who

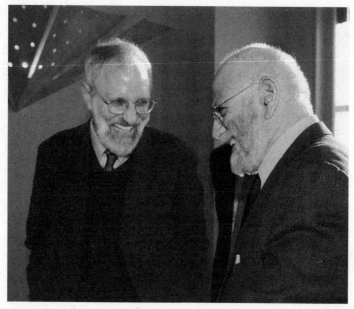

Ken Kendler (left) and Oliver Sacks at a reception in New York City in 2008. (Courtesy of Eve Vagg, New York State Psychiatric Institute)

saw mental illness through a narrow theoretical lens and proclaimed their approach the only valid one. Their exclusionary approach to psychiatry reflects what Kendler calls "epistemic hubris." The best antidote for this hubris, observes Kendler, is an evidence-based pluralism.

Eric Kandel is justly famous for his role in launching the brain revolution in psychiatry; the full sweep of his career reflects a pluralistic vision of mental illness. While Kandel's research focused on unraveling the neurobiology of memory, it was motivated and framed by his belief in the psychodynamic theories of Freud. He never relinquished his guiding faith that even if some of Freud's specific ideas were wrong, the psychodynamic perspective on the mind was as necessary and valuable as the biological perspective. Kandel's pluralism was reflected in a seminal paper he published in 1979 in the *New*

England Journal of Medicine entitled "Psychotherapy and the Single Synapse." In the paper, Kandel observed that psychiatrists tended to fall into two types—the "hard-nosed" psychiatrists who yearned for biological explanations of disorders, and the "soft-nosed" psychiatrists who believed that biology had delivered little of practical use and that the future of psychiatry lay in the development of new psychotherapies. Then Kandel observed that this apparent tension in perspectives could actually be a source of future progress, as the two sides were forced to contend and eventually reconcile with each other. Kandel still maintains his pluralistic perspective today, as seen in his 2013 *New York Times* op-ed, written in response to David Brooks's critique of the *DSM-5*:

> This new science of the mind is based on the principle that our mind and our brain are inseparable. The brain is responsible not only for relatively simple motor behaviors like running and eating, but also for complex acts that we consider quintessentially human, like thinking, speaking, and creating works of art. Looked at from this perspective, our mind is a set of operations carried out by our brain. The same principle of unity applies to mental disorders.

So after all is said and done, what *is* mental illness? We know that mental disorders exhibit consistent clusters of symptoms. We know that many disorders feature distinctive neural signatures in the brain. We know that many disorders express distinctive patterns of brain activity. We have gained some insight into the genetic underpinnings of mental disorders. We can treat persons with mental disorders using medications and somatic therapies that act uniquely on their symptoms but exert no effects in healthy people. We know that specific types of psychotherapy lead to clear improvements in patients suffering from specific types of disorders. And we know that, left untreated, these disorders cause anguish, misery, disability, violence, even death. Thus, mental disorders are abnormal, enduring, harmful, treatable, feature a biological component, and can be reliably diagnosed. I believe this should satisfy anyone's definition of medical illness.

At the same time, mental disorders represent a form of medical illness unlike any other. The brain is the only organ that can suffer what we might call "existential disease"—where its operation is disrupted not by physical injury but by impalpable experience. Every other organ in the body requires a physical stimulus to generate illness—toxins, infections, blunt force trauma, strangulation—but only the brain can become ill from such incorporeal stimuli as loneliness, humiliation, or fear. Getting fired from a job or being abandoned by a spouse can induce depression. Watching your child get run over by a car or losing your retirement savings in a financial crisis may cause PTSD. The brain is an interface between the ethereal and the organic, where the feelings and memories composing the ineffable fabric of experience are transmuted into molecular biochemistry. Mental illness is a medical condition—but it's also an existential condition. Within this peculiar duality lies all the historic tumult and future promise of my profession— as well as our species' consuming fascination with human behavior and mental illness.

No matter how advanced our biological assays, brain-imaging technologies, and genetic capabilities become, I doubt they will ever fully replace the psychodynamic element that is inherent in existential disease. Interpretation of the highly personal human element of mental illness by a compassionate physician will always be an essential part of psychiatry, even in the case of the most biological of mental illnesses, such as Autism Spectrum Disorders and Alzheimer's disease. At the same time, a purely psychodynamic account of a patient's disorder will never suffice to account for the underlying neural and physiological aberrations giving rise to the manifest symptoms. Only by combining a sensitive awareness of a patient's experiential state with all the available biological data can psychiatrists hope to offer the most effective care.

While I am deeply sympathetic to Tom Insel's position—I, too, certainly want to see an improved neurobiological understanding of mental illnesses—I believe that psychiatry is served best when we resist the lure of epistemic hubris and remain open to evidence and ideas from multiple perspectives. The *DSM-5* is neither a botched attempt at a biological psychiatry nor a throwback to psychodynamic constructs, but rather an unbridled triumph of pluralism. After Insel posted his incendiary blog, I called him to discuss the situation, and together we ultimately agreed to issue a joint statement from the APA and the NIMH to reassure patients, providers, and payers that the *DSM-5* was still the accepted standard for clinical care—at least until additional scientific progress justified its upgrade or replacement.

Since the *DSM-5*'s launch in May 2013, an amazing thing has occurred. There has been a deafening silence from critics and the media. It now appears that the controversy and uproar before its release was focused on the perceived *process* of creating the *DSM-5* as well as on an effort to influence the actual content that made it into the published version. And in the aftermath, while many critics in and out of psychiatry have expressed understandable disappointment about "what might have been"—what if the APA had appointed different leadership, what if the process had been managed differently, and what if other criteria than those officially adopted define a given disorder—it has been gratifyingly clear that health care providers and consumers have been well served by the *DSM-5*.

But the far-ranging and heated conflict that played out

online and in the media did make one thing salient: Psychiatry has become deeply ingrained within the fabric of our culture, winding through our most prominent social institutions and coloring our most mundane daily encounters. For better or worse, the *DSM* is not merely a compendium of medical diagnoses. It has become a public document that helps define how we understand ourselves and how we live our lives.

Chapter 10

The End of Stigma: The Future of Psychiatry

We need our families and friends to understand that the 100 mil-lion Americans suffering with mental illness are not lost souls or lost causes. We're fully capable of getting better, being happy, and building rewarding relationships.
— Congressman Patrick J. Kennedy, on his diagnosis of
bipolar disorder

How come every other organ in your body can get sick and you get sympathy, except the brain?
— Ruby Wax

Hidden in the Attic

I've been fortunate to live through the most dramatic and posi-tive sea change in the history of my medical specialty, as it matured from a psychoanalytic cult of shrinks into a scientific medicine of the brain.

Four decades ago, when my cousin Catherine needed treat-ment for her mental illness, I steered her away from the most prominent and well-established psychiatric facilities of the time, fearing they might only make things worse. Today, I wouldn't hesitate to send her to the psychiatric department of any major medical center. As someone who has worked in the front-line trenches of clinical care and at the top echelons of psychiatric research, I've seen firsthand the sweeping progress that has transformed psychiatry... but, sadly, not everyone has been able to benefit from this progress.

Shortly after I became chair of psychiatry at Columbia University, I was asked to consult on a sixty-six-year-old woman named Mrs. Kim. She had been admitted to our hospital with a very severe skin infection that seemed to have gone untreated for a long time. This was puzzling, because Mrs. Kim was both educated and affluent. She had graduated from medical school and as the wife of a prominent Asian industrialist she had access to the very best health care.

As I spoke with Mrs. Kim, I quickly discovered why a psychiatrist had been called to see a patient with a skin infection. When I tried to ask how she was feeling, she began to shout incoherently and make bizarre, angry gestures. When I remained silent and unobtrusively observed her, she talked to herself—or, more accurately, she talked to nonexistent people. Since I could not engage her in conversation, I decided to speak with her family. The next day, her husband and adult son and daughter reluctantly came to my office. After a great deal of cajoling, they revealed that shortly after Mrs. Kim graduated from medical school, she had developed symptoms of schizophrenia.

Her family was ashamed of her condition. Despite their wealth and resources, neither Mrs. Kim's parents nor her husband sought any kind of treatment for her illness; instead, they decided to do whatever they could to prevent anyone from discovering her ignominious diagnosis. They sectioned off her living quarters in a wing of their spacious home and kept her isolated whenever they had guests. Despite her having received a medical degree, practicing medicine was completely out of the question. Mrs. Kim rarely left the property and never for any extended period of time—until she developed the skin rash. Her family tried all kinds of over-the-counter remedies hoping that they would take care of the problem. But when it became infected and rapidly began to spread, they became frightened and called the family doctor. When he saw her torso dotted with purulent abscesses, he implored the family to take her to the hospital, where she was diagnosed with a severe staph infection.

Stunned, I repeated back to them what they had just told me—that for the past thirty-some years, they had conspired together to keep their wife and mother shut off from the world to avoid public embarrassment. They unabashedly nodded their heads in unison. I was incredulous—this was something out of a Charlotte Brontë novel rather than twenty-first-century New York City. I told them quite bluntly that their decision to withhold treatment was both cruel and immoral—though, tragically, not illegal—and I urged them to let us transfer her to the psychiatric unit of the hospital so that she could be treated. After some skeptical discussion, they refused.

They informed me that even if Mrs. Kim could be successfully treated, at this point the resulting changes would be too disruptive to their lives and their position in the community. They would have to explain to friends and acquaintances the reason Mrs. Kim suddenly began to appear in public after such a long absence—and who knows what Mrs. Kim herself might say or how she would behave in such circumstances? The Kims perceived the stigma of mental illness as so daunting that they would rather have this once intelligent, otherwise physically healthy woman remain psychotic and incapacitated, her brain irreversibly deteriorating, than face the social consequences of acknowledging her mental illness.

A few short generations ago, the greatest obstacles to the treatment of mental illness were the lack of effective treatments, unreliable diagnostic criteria, and an ossified theory of the basic nature of the disease. Today the single greatest hindrance to treatment is not any gap in scientific knowledge or shortcoming in medical capability but the social stigma. This stigma, unfortunately, has been sustained by the legacy of psychiatry's historic failures and its enduring reputation—no longer justified—as the unwanted stepchild of medicine.

Though we live in a time of unprecedented tolerance of different races, religions, and sexual orientations, mental illness—an involuntary medical condition that affects one out of four people—is still regarded as a mark of shame, a scarlet letter C for "crazy," P for "psycho," or M for "mental." Imagine you were invited to a friend's wedding but unexpectedly came down with an illness. Would you prefer to say that you had to cancel because of a kidney stone...or a manic episode? Would you rather offer as your excuse that you threw out your back... or suffered a panic attack? Would you rather explain that you were having a migraine...or were hung over from having gone on a bender?

I encounter evidence of this shame and sensitivity nearly every day. Many of the patients seen by our faculty prefer to pay out of pocket rather than use their health insurance, for fear of their psychiatric treatment becoming known. Other patients choose not to come to see our doctors in the Columbia *Psychiatry* Clinic or visit me in the New York State *Psychiatric* Institute, preferring a private medical office without any signs indicating the identity of the medical specialty inside. Patients frequently fly here to New York from South America, the Middle East, or Asia to consult with us just to make sure nobody from their country finds out that they're consulting a psychiatrist.

A few years ago, I gave a talk at a luncheon in midtown Manhattan about mental illness to raise funds for psychiatry research. Afterwards, I circulated among the attendees— smart, successful, and outgoing people who had all been personally invited to the event by Sarah Foster, a prominent socialite whose schizophrenic son had committed suicide some years ago while a senior in high school. They chatted over poached salmon and Chablis, openly praising Sarah's selfless efforts to raise awareness about mental illness—though none of them admitted any direct experience with mental illness themselves. Instead, mental illness was treated like the genocide in Sudan or the tsunami in Indonesia: an issue highly deserving of public attention, but one quite distant and removed from the patrons' own lives.

Several days later, I received a call at my office. One of the attendees, an editor at a publishing company, asked if I could help her. It seemed that she had lost interest in her job, had trouble sleeping, and frequently become very emotional, even tearful. Was she having a midlife crisis? I agreed to see her, and eventually diagnosed her as suffering from depression. But before she made the appointment with me, she insisted I keep it completely confidential—and added, "Please don't say anything to Sarah!"

The very next day I got a call from another attendee. This woman worked at a private equity firm and was concerned because her twenty-something son had dropped out of graduate school to start his own company. Though she admired his entrepreneurial spirit, his grandiose idea for a new software application to end world poverty was conceived during a period of erratic and sleepless behavior. After evaluating her son, my initial suspicion was confirmed: He was in the incipient stages of a manic episode.

Over the next few weeks, I received more calls from Sarah's invitees seeking help for spouses with addictions, siblings with anxiety, parents with dementia, young children with attentional problems, and adult children still living at home. Over time, fully half of the people who attended Sarah's luncheon reached out to me, including the owner of the restaurant where the event was held.

These were all educated and sophisticated people with access to the very best health care money could buy. If they had trouble breathing or suffered a prolonged fever, they likely would have obtained help from their personal physicians, or at least sought out the best possible referral. Yet because of the stigma of mental illness, they had avoided seeking medical attention for their issues until they fortuitously met a psychiatrist at a fund-raiser for mental illness. And amazingly, even though they had been invited to the fund-raiser by a friend who devoted herself to raising awareness about mental illness after the tragedy of her son's death, none of them wanted Sarah to know about their own problem.

It's finally time to end this stigma—and, now, there is good reason to think we can.

Bridging the Gap

Receiving a diagnosis of mental illness can scar your self-image as if the doctor has seared an ignominious brand onto your forehead for all the world to see—every bit as pernicious as the historic stigmas affixed to other medical conditions once considered loathsome, such as epilepsy, leprosy, smallpox, cancer, and AIDS (and more recently, Ebola). In times past, victims of these maladies were shunned as pariahs. Yet in each case, scientific advances eventually revealed the true nature of the illnesses, and society came to understand that it was neither a moral failing nor a divine scourge. Once medical science discovered the causes and began to deliver effective treatments for these diseases, the stigma began to dissipate. Today, we've reached a point where players in the National Football League wear pink during games to express support for victims of breast cancer, every major city has a fund-raising walk for AIDS research, and we have a national autism awareness day. This dramatic shift in public attitudes came about as people began to talk openly about stigmatized conditions—and, perhaps most important, began to have faith in medicine's ability to understand and treat them.

Our first real opportunity to eliminate the stigma shrouding mental illness has finally arrived because most mental illnesses can be diagnosed and treated very effectively. Yet the stigma has persisted because the public has not become aware of psychiatry's advances in the same swift way that it became aware of advances in heart disease, cancer, and AIDS treatment. Or, perhaps more to the point, the public does not yet *believe* that psychiatry has truly advanced.

Today, psychiatrists are well integrated with the rest of medicine and approach mental illness as they do any other medical disorder. They may prescribe medication or apply ECT to treat a disorder, while simultaneously providing proven forms of psychotherapy. They may recommend evidence-based changes in diet, sleep, exercise, or lifestyle to reduce the risk of developing an illness or to reduce its effects. They communicate openly and frequently with other medical specialists, and they may delegate some components of a patient's treatment to allied mental health professionals, such as psychologists, social workers, psychiatric nurses, and rehabilitation therapists. They engage with their patients in a direct and empathic manner. And they get good results.

Contemporary psychiatrists hold a pluralistic view of mental illness that embraces neuroscience, psychopharmacology, and genetics—but also wields psychotherapy and psychosocial techniques in order to understand patients' unique histories and treat their conditions in an individualized way.

In the past, it was widely believed that medical students went into psychiatry to solve their own problems, a conviction espoused even within the medical profession. And it's true psychiatry sometimes ended up as the safety net for medical students who were too weak to compete in other disciplines—as it still remains in some Asian and Middle Eastern countries to this day. But times have changed.

Psychiatry now competes with other medical specialties for the top trainees. In 2010, we were trying to recruit a talented MD/PhD named Mohsin Ahmed, who was considering applying to the Columbia psychiatry program. He had completed his PhD in neurobiology under a celebrated neuroscientist who proclaimed him one of the most talented graduate students he ever had. Ahmed was a prized recruit and had his pick of any program in the country. Although he had signaled his interest in psychiatry, it was clear he harbored some reservations.

I made it a point to talk with Ahmed on several occasions during his interviews and did my best to convey the excitement in my field—how it was being transformed by neuroscience while still enabling its practitioners to maintain personal involvement with patients. When the results of the annual process of matching graduating medical students with training programs came out, I was thrilled to see that he had selected psychiatry after all and was coming to Columbia. But midway through his first year, he started having second thoughts about his choice of specialties and told our training director he wanted to switch to neurology.

I promptly arranged to meet with him. He told me he was fascinated by the daunting complexities of mental illnesses but disappointed by the clinical practice of psychiatry. "We still base diagnoses on symptoms, and assess the effectiveness of treatments by observing the patient rather than relying on laboratory measures," Ahmed lamented. "I want to feel like I have some real sense of why my patients are sick and what our treatments are doing in their brains to help them."

How could I argue with him? Ahmed's concerns were a common refrain—echoed by everyone from Wilhelm Griesinger to Tom Insel—and were entirely valid. But I explained that even though we were still bridging the gap between psychological constructs and neurobiological mechanisms, it was entirely possible to embrace both, as Eric Kandel, Ken Kendler, and many other world-class psychiatric researchers have done. The most exciting psychiatry research in the twenty-first century is linked to neuroscience, and all the leaders in our field now have some kind of biological or neurological training. At the same time, there is still steady progress in psychotherapy. Cognitive-behavioral therapy, one of the most effective forms of psychotherapy for depression, has recently been adapted by psychodynamic pioneer Aaron Beck to treat the negative symptoms of patients with schizophrenia—a remarkable achievement at any age, but a stunning accomplishment for an indefatigable researcher in his nineties.

I told Ahmed that his generation would be the one to finally close the gap between psychodynamic constructs and biological mechanisms—and given his own abilities and passions, he could lead the way. Ahmed is now one of our top psychiatry trainees and is conducting an innovative project on the pathophysiology of psychotic disorders. Ironically, despite maintaining his focus on neuroscience research, he has shown himself to be a most empathic and skilled psychotherapist, with a real knack for connecting with patients. To my mind, he personifies the twenty-first-century psychiatrist. No longer an alienist, shrink, pill-pusher, or reductionist neuroscientist, Mohsin Ahmed has become a compassionate and pluralistic psychiatric physician.

From Psycho to Silver Linings

Now that the field of psychiatry has acquired the scientific knowledge and clinical capability to manage mental illness effectively and is attracting some of the best and the brightest talent into the profession, changing popular culture and society's attitudes toward psychiatry and mental illness has become the final, and perhaps most challenging, task of all.

The Hollywood stereotype of the homicidal maniac was indelibly emblazoned in the public's mind by the 1960 Alfred

Hitchcock film *Psycho*. The protagonist, Norman Bates, is a psychotic motel proprietor who channels his deceased mother in drag before viciously murdering his guests. Needless to say, this lurid fictional portrayal wildly exaggerates clinical reality. But ever since *Psycho*'s commercial success, there has been a parade of psychotic murderers in cinema, from *Halloween*'s Michael Myers to *Nightmare on Elm Street*'s Freddy Krueger to *Saw*'s Jigsaw.

The motion picture industry also has a long tradition of portraying psychiatrists and other mental health workers as weird, ignorant, or cruel, starting with such films as *Shock* (1946) and *The Snake Pit* (1948), which depict the horrors of asylums, and continuing through *One Flew Over the Cuckoo's Nest*, *The Silence of the Lambs* (featuring a manipulative, arrogant director of a mental institution), *Girl, Interrupted* (featuring a mental ward for young women where the staff are oblivious to the true problems of their patients), *Gothika* (featuring a creepy mental institution with a sadistic, murderous director), *Shutter Island* (featuring a creepy mental institution with staff who appear manipulative, arrogant, and violent), *Side Effects* (featuring manipulative psychiatrists and greedy pharmaceutical companies), and even *Terminator 2* (portraying the staff of a mental hospital as cold and foolish rather than compassionate and competent).

But in recent years, Hollywood has begun to present another side of mental illness. Ron Howard's film *A Beautiful Mind* tells the moving story of economist John Nash, who suffered from schizophrenia yet went on to win the Nobel Prize. Another example is the hit TV series *Homeland*, featuring a brilliant CIA analyst (played by Claire Danes) who suffers from bipolar disorder and is supported by her smart, caring psychiatrist sister. Apart from the interesting plot and fine acting, the series is remarkable for its authentic and accurate portrayal of both the effects of the protagonist's mental disorder and its treatment—while showing that mental illness need not limit someone from attaining a high level of professional competence.

The Best Picture–nominated *Silver Linings Playbook* offered a realistic portrayal of appealing characters with mental disorders. They live purposeful lives in which their illnesses do not define them but instead are merely part of the fabric of their lives. When Jennifer Lawrence accepted her Best Actress Oscar for her role in the movie, she proclaimed, "If you have asthma you take asthma medicine. If you have diabetes you take diabetes medicine. But as soon as you have to take medicine for your brain, you are immediately stigmatized."

Lawrence's co-star, Bradley Cooper, who played a young man regaining his balance after a destructive bout of bipolar disorder, became an advocate for mental illness after the role. I'll never forget what Cooper told me at a White House Conference on Mental Health in 2013, when I asked what motivated his advocacy. "Working on the film reminded me of an old friend who I knew in high school and was mentally ill. It dawned on me what he had been dealing with, and made me feel ashamed of how I offered him no support or understanding, only ignorance and indifference. Making this film made me wonder how many other people out there are similarly unaware as I was and that I can help bring them the same awareness that the film brought me."

The actress Glenn Close embodies Hollywood's improving attitude toward mental illness. Twenty-five years ago, she gave a riveting performance as a pet-killing, homicidal character with borderline personality disorder in *Fatal Attraction*. Today, Close has emerged as the most visible spokesperson for mental illness in the entertainment industry. She started the Bring Change 2 Mind nonprofit, whose mission is "to end the stigma and discrimination surrounding mental illness." Close travels the country educating people about psychiatric research and treatments for mental illness. Her motivation is her family: Her sister Jessie suffers from bipolar disorder and her nephew Calen has schizoaffective disorder.

Numerous celebrities have been willing to talk openly about their own experience with mental illness. The mega-selling author Danielle Steel started a foundation to commemorate her son Nick Traina, who committed suicide after battling bipolar disorder. Talk show host Dick Cavett and *60 Minutes* anchor Mike Wallace bravely spoke out about their struggles with depression. Catherine Zeta-Jones revealed her hospitalization for bipolar disorder. Kitty Dukakis, wife of presidential candidate Michael Dukakis, wrote a book about the life-saving role of ECT in controlling her depression.

I have had the good fortune to become personally acquainted with Jane Pauley as the result of her own experience and public advocacy for mental illness. The former *Today* show anchor writes about the role bipolar disorder has played in her life in her books *Skywriting* and *Your Life Calling*. She recounts how in the small Indiana town where she grew up, no one knew about mental illness, much less talked about it. As a result, she never gave her frequent mood changes much thought, until she landed in the psychiatric ward at the age of fifty-one after a course of the steroid medication prednisone triggered a severe manic episode. This unexpected hospitalization finally compelled Pauley to come to grips with the suppressed history of mood disorders in her family—and the fact that she had unknowingly endured the symptoms of bipolar disorder for years. She could have chosen to keep her condition private, but instead Jane made the brave decision to speak out about it.

Other celebrities provoke public discussion of the stigma of mental illness only after they succumb to its effects. At the age of sixty-three, Robin Williams, one of the most talented comedians of his generation—famed for his frenetic, high-octane brand of humor—tried to slash his wrist, then hanged himself in his bedroom with a belt. Fans were shocked to discover that a man who shared so much joy and passion with the world had apparently struggled with severe depression most of his life. While his tragic suicide is an immeasurable loss, it was at least reassuring to find that most of the media coverage invited mental health professionals to address head-on the apparent paradox of a man who seemed to be so loved simultaneously feeling he had nothing to live for.

In another indication of how cultural attitudes are changing, a scion of America's most famous political family has emerged as a passionate spokesperson for mental illness. Patrick Joseph Kennedy is the youngest child of Massachusetts senator Edward Kennedy and the nephew of President John F. Kennedy. He was the youngest member of the Kennedy family to hold political office when, at the age of twenty-one, he was elected to the Rhode Island House of Representatives in 1988. He was elected to Congress in 1994.

I first met Patrick at a fund-raiser held at a friend's home in 2006. Though he was still in Congress, his admirable legislative record had become overshadowed by stories of intoxication and emotional instability. The previous May he'd crashed his car into a barricade on Capitol Hill. Shortly afterward, he went to the Mayo Clinic for detox and rehab. When I met him, despite his voluble and engaging political persona, he seemed a bit shaky and disjointed—symptoms of his bipolar disorder, I assumed.

Five years later, I encountered Patrick again at a meeting on mental health care in Washington, DC, and I was struck by how much he had changed. He was composed, focused, and responsive. When I inquired about this apparent change, he explained that he had received effective treatment for his bipolar disorder and substance abuse and was living a healthy lifestyle and feeling great. A year later I attended his engagement party in New York. After the toasts and congratulatory comments, Patrick pulled me aside and informed me that he had decided to devote the next phase of his career to being an advocate for mental illness and addictions.

Inspired by his decision, I made up my mind to run for the APA presidency the very next day. If I was fortunate enough to win, I thought Patrick would be the perfect partner in my own mission to eliminate the stigma associated with mental illness and educate people about psychiatry. Since then, Patrick and I have worked together on many psychiatry-related legislative initiatives, including the Final Rule of the Mental Health Parity and Addiction Equity Act, the Patient Protection and Affordable Care Act, and the Helping Families in Mental Health Crisis Act. We have also joined efforts to communicate the true state of affairs about mental illness, addiction, and

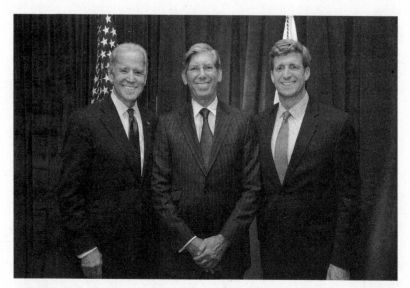

Former congressman Patrick Kennedy (right) with Vice President Joseph Biden and the author at the 50th Anniversary of the Community Mental Health Act at the JFK Presidential Library in Boston, October 25, 2013. (Ellen Dallager Photography, American Psychiatric Association, 2014)

mental health care to the public. Patrick has become perhaps the most visible, articulate, and effective spokesperson for mental illness in America—and the first politician to confront his own serious mental illness in such a public and positive manner.

Patrick Kennedy, along with Bradley Cooper, Glenn Close, and Jane Pauley, is joined by many other celebrities, including Alan Alda, Goldie Hawn, and Arianna Huffington, who are all beginning to use their visibility and influence to raise awareness about mental illness. This is a good start, but the truth is that we will only overcome the stigma of mental illness when the public is fully convinced that medical science understands mental illness and can provide effective treatment. Fortunately, even more impressive developments in psychiatry are just around the corner.

A Bright Future

Over the past two hundred years, the history of psychiatry has been characterized by long stretches of stagnation punctuated by abrupt and transformative changes—many of which, regrettably, were not for the better. But we have entered a period of scientific advances that will produce a stream of innovations more dazzling than any that have come before.

One of the most promising arenas of research is genetics. It is virtually certain that no single gene alone is responsible for any particular mental illness, but through increasingly powerful genetic techniques we are starting to understand how certain patterns or networks of genes confer levels of risk. These genetic signatures will lead to more precise diagnosis of patients. They will also permit earlier identification of persons vulnerable to severe mental illness, enabling preventive interventions.

Glenn Close's family provided one of the first examples of

the application of genetics in psychiatry. In 2011, her sister Jessie and nephew Calen volunteered for a research study at McLean Hospital in Massachusetts led by Dr. Deborah Levy, a psychologist at Harvard. A genetic analysis of Jessie and Calen's DNA (using ROMA-like methods) revealed that they shared a rare genetic variant resulting in extra copies of the gene that produces an enzyme that metabolizes the amino acid glycine, which has been implicated in psychotic disorders (as it helps to modulate the activity of the excitatory neurotransmitter glutamate). Extra copies of this gene meant that Jessie and Calen were deficient in glycine, since their body overproduced the enzyme that metabolized glycine. When Dr. Levy gave them supplemental glycine, Jessie and Calen's psychiatric symptoms markedly improved. It was like watching a patient's fever decline after giving him aspirin. When they stopped taking the supplemental glycine, their symptoms worsened.

Using a genetic test on Glenn Close's sister and nephew in order to identify a specific drug that could ameliorate their mental illness was one of the very first applications of personalized medicine in psychiatry. It holds the promise of revolutionizing the diagnosis and treatment of mental illness.

I believe we will soon have useful diagnostic tests for mental illness. In addition to the progress made toward genetic tests, there are several other promising technologies that could lead to tests that can aid in diagnosis and treatment selection, including electrophysiology (establishing an EKG-like test of brain activity), serology (which would produce a blood test similar to the tests for cholesterol or prostate-specific antigen), and brain imaging (using MRI and PET procedures to detect signature brain structures and activity). The FDA recently approved PET testing for Alzheimer's disease, and we are getting very close to using brain imaging to aid in the diagnosis of autism. Then, instead of Daniel Amen's spurious claims for SPECT-based diagnosis of mental illness, we will have scientifically proven methods of diagnosis using brain-imaging procedures.

Advances in psychiatric treatment are also occurring on other fronts. New drugs are being developed that are more precisely targeted in terms of where and how they act within the brain. Brain stimulation therapy (the treatment modality that began as ECT) is also undergoing remarkable progress. Researchers have devised two new forms of brain stimulation that are much less invasive than ECT: transcranial magnetic stimulation (TMS) and transcranial direct-current stimulation (TDCS). These therapies use magnetic fields or weak electrical current to stimulate or dampen brain activity in specific anatomic regions without inducing a seizure, and they are noninvasive and don't require anesthesia. They can be used to target specific brain sites believed to be the source of symptoms of psychosis, depression, and anxiety.

For the most severe and intractable mental illnesses that don't respond to medications or other forms of brain stimulation therapy, deep brain stimulation (DBS) offers new hope. DBS involves surgically implanting an electrode into a precisely defined neural structure. While this procedure is highly invasive and requires neurosurgery, as a treatment of last resort it has been used successfully to treat extreme cases of obsessive-compulsive disorder and depression, as well as neurological disorders like Parkinson's disease and torsion dystonia.

One encouraging avenue of psychotherapy research is coming out of cognitive neuroscience, a field that studies the software of the brain. This work is beginning to elucidate the neural bases of mental functions that can be modified through talk therapy—and mental functions *not* amenable to talk therapy. We are starting to understand the specific neurobiological processes that are active during psychotherapy and can use this information to refine psychotherapy techniques, applying them only to conditions that they are most likely to help.

Other researchers are combining specific medications with talk therapy to enhance its efficacy. Antidepressants, antipsychotics, and anxiolytics are frequently used to reduce symptoms that interfere with a patient's ability to benefit from talk therapy—it's hard to meaningfully engage when you are having psychotic thoughts or hearing screaming voices, severely depressed, or paralyzed by anxiety. Drugs that enhance learning and neuroplasticity can increase the effectiveness of psychotherapy and reduce the number of sessions necessary to produce change.

One example of such synergistic effects is combining cognitive-behavioral therapy with D-cycloserine, a drug initially approved for the treatment of tuberculosis. Scientists have learned that D-cycloserine enhanced learning by acting on glutamate receptors in the brain. When D-cycloserine is used with cognitive-behavioral therapy, it appears to enhance its effects. Similar joint drug-psychotherapy treatments have also been successfully applied to patients with obsessive-compulsive disorder, anxiety disorders, and PTSD.

Another recent example came from the lab of my colleague Scott Small, a neurologist at Columbia University. Small found that a concentrated extract of flavanols from cocoa beans dramatically enhanced the memory of people with age-associated memory impairment by stimulating neural activity in the hippocampus. Such neutraceutical compounds may provide a new approach to cognitive rehabilitation.

We are also seeing the start of a flood of Internet-based applications for mobile devices that assist patients with treatment adherence, provide auxiliary therapeutic support, and enable patients to remain in virtual contact with their mental health providers. David Kimhy, the director of the Experimental Psychopathology Laboratory at Columbia University, developed a mobile app that schizophrenic patients can use when they are in distress. If their auditory hallucinations intensify, they can launch a cognitive-behavioral script on their smart phone that instructs them how to cope with their symptoms:

> Screen 1: Do you hear voices right now? [Yes / No]
> Screen 2: How strong is the voice? [1–100 scale]
> Screen 3: What would you like to do?
>> Relaxation Exercise
>> Pleasurable Activities
>> Explore Causes
>> Nothing
> Screen 4.1: <u>Relaxation Exercise</u>: *[Run on-screen guided breathing exercise for 45 seconds]*

Richard Sloan, director of Behavioral Medicine of Columbia Psychiatry, monitors bio-signals (including heart rate, blood pressure, respiration, temperature, muscle tension) of patients by having them wear accouterments ranging from wrist bands to vests tricked out with sensors that transmit data in real time, thereby providing a virtual display of a person's emotional state.

Psychiatry has come a long way since the days of chaining lunatics in cold stone cells and parading them as freakish marvels in front of a gaping public. After a difficult and often disreputable journey, my profession now practices an enlightened and effective medicine of mental health, giving rise to the most gratifying moments in a psychiatrist's career: bearing witness to clinical triumphs. Often, these are not merely the relief of a patient's symptoms but the utter transformation of a person's life.

A few years back I had a patient like Abigail Abercrombie who suffered from panic attacks and had been homebound for two decades. At first, I had to make house calls just to see her, since she refused to leave the dismal safety of her cramped Manhattan apartment. When she was finally able to visit me at my office, she sat near the open door with her bicycle perched just outside so she could flee at any moment. Today, she goes hiking with her husband, socializes with friends, and takes her children to school, telling me, "I feel like my world has become a hundred times larger."

I treated a fifty-year-old man who suffered from a nearly lifelong depression and twice tried to kill himself. He quit several jobs and was unable to maintain a romantic relationship. After two months of treatment with antidepressant medication and psychotherapy, he felt that a veil of gloom had been lifted and asked, "Is this how most people feel? Is this how most people *live?*"

My friend Andrew Solomon also suffered from suicidal depression for years before receiving effective treatment. He wrote eloquently about his illness in *The Noonday Demon: An Atlas of Depression,* a Pulitzer Prize finalist and winner of the National Book Award. Today, he is happily married and enjoys a very successful career as a writer, activist, and highly prized speaker. "Without modern psychiatry," Solomon assures me, "I truly believe I might have been dead by now."

Not so very long ago, those suffering from bipolar disorder, such as Patrick Kennedy, had every reason to believe that their lives would inexorably lead to financial ruin, public humiliation, and wrecked relationships. Kay Jamison, another dear friend, was whipsawed between careening flights of mania and crushing bouts of depression when she was a graduate student and junior faculty member in psychology at UCLA. Her prospects looked bleak. Today she is a tenured professor of psychiatry at Johns Hopkins and was named a "Hero of Medicine" and one of the "Best Doctors in the United States" by *Time* magazine. Her writing, including five books, is highly acclaimed and earned her an honorary doctor of letters from the University of St. Andrews. She says psychiatry "restored her life."

What about the most severe and frightening of psychiatry's flagship illnesses, the supreme scourge of the mind: schizophrenia? Today, if a person with schizophrenia, the most virulent form of psychosis, comes to the psychiatry department of a major medical center and fully avails herself of quality treatment—and sticks with it after she is discharged—the most likely outcome is recovery and the ability to have an independent life and continue her education or career. Consider my friend Elyn Saks.

She grew up in an upper-middle-class family in Miami, where she enjoyed the love of her parents and the sunny comforts of a Norman Rockwell–like childhood. Though in retrospect there may have been a few clues about her mental illness to come—when Elyn was eight, she would not go to bed until all her shoes and books had been carefully arranged in unvarying and precise order, and she often hauled the covers over her head because some menacing figure was lurking outside her bedroom window—any casual visitor to the Saks home would have found a happy, intelligent, and perfectly normal little girl. It was not till she went to college, at Vanderbilt University in Nashville, that her behavior began to change.

At first, Elyn's hygiene deteriorated. She stopped showering regularly and often wore the same clothes day after day till her friends told her to change them. After that, her activities grew downright disturbing. On one occasion she bolted from her dorm room for no discernible reason, abandoning a friend who was visiting her from Miami, and dashed around the quad in the freezing cold waving a blanket over her head and declaring for all to hear that she could fly. However, these foreboding signs failed to elicit treatment for her, nor did they prevent her from graduating as class valedictorian and winning a Marshall scholarship to study in England at Oxford University.

In England she experienced her first psychotic breakdown. She describes this episode in her award-winning book *The*

Center Cannot Hold: My Journey Through Madness: "I was unable to sleep, a mantra running through my head: I am a piece of shit and I deserve to die. I am a piece of shit and I deserve to die. I am a piece of shit and I deserve to die. Time stopped. By the middle of the night, I was convinced day would never come again. The thoughts of death were all around me."

She was hospitalized with the diagnosis of schizophrenia, yet—this being 1983—she was treated mainly with talk therapy. No medication was prescribed for her.

After she was released, she somehow completed her studies at Oxford and was even admitted to Yale Law School, but her illness worsened. In New Haven, Elyn started to believe that people were reading her mind and attempting to control her movements and behavior. Moreover, her thoughts were disjointed and bizarre, and when she spoke she was barely coherent. One afternoon she visited the office of her contracts professor, a smart, funny woman whom Elyn liked and idealized because "she's God and I will bask in her God-like glow." When Elyn arrived, looking and acting strange, the professor informed her that she was concerned about her and suggested that Elyn come home with her as soon as she finished up some work in her office. Delighted, Elyn promptly jumped to her feet and climbed out the window onto the ledge. Rocking and kicking her feet, she began belting out Beethoven's "Ode to Joy." Elyn was hospitalized again, this time against her will, and was placed in physical restraints and forcibly medicated.

Elyn told me that this was the worst experience of her life, the moment when it really sank in that she was mentally ill—suffering from incurable, perpetual, mind-warping schizophrenia. She felt sure she would never have a normal life. "I thought I would need to reduce the scope of my dreams," she said. "Sometimes I just wanted to be dead." But in New Haven, she encountered a pluralistic psychiatrist ("Dr. White," in her memoirs) —a Freudian psychoanalyst who embraced the therapeutic power of psychopharmaceuticals—who provided her with both structure and hope by talking with her each and every day while waiting for her medication to take hold and continuing thereafter. She eventually was placed on clozapine, a new antipsychotic drug with superior therapeutic powers, approved for use in the U.S. in 1989.

Encouraged by Dr. White, Elyn decided that she would not let her illness dictate her fate. She began learning everything she could about schizophrenia and diligently participated in all of her treatments. Before long, she was functioning well and living a clear-headed life once again. She believes her family's, and subsequently her husband's, unwavering love and support were essential to her success, and having met them, I wholeheartedly concur.

Supported by her loved ones and by a pluralistic psychiatry, Elyn has gone on to enjoy an extraordinary career as a legal scholar, mental health advocate, and author. Today she is an associate dean and professor of law, psychology, psychiatry, and the behavioral sciences at the University of Southern California. She won a MacArthur "Genius" award and recently gave a TED talk urging compassion for those with mental illness, recognizing the importance of human empathy in her own recovery, and wrote her bestselling book.

Elyn Saks, Kay Jamison, and Andrew Solomon didn't just have their symptoms alleviated. With the aid of effective, scientifically based, compassionate, and caring treatment, they were able to discover entirely new identities within themselves. This was an impossible dream a century ago and was not the norm even thirty years ago, at the start of my medical career. Today, recovery is not just possible, but expected. A self-determined, fulfilling life is the goal for all people with mental illness.

However, despite this progress and the proliferation of auspicious developments in our society's understanding of mental illness and psychiatry, I am under no illusion that the specters of psychiatry's past have vanished, or that my profession has freed itself from suspicion and scorn. Rather, I believe that after a long and tumultuous journey, psychiatry has arrived at a pivotal and propitious moment in its evolution — a moment well worth celebrating, but also an opportunity to reflect on the work that still lies ahead. In doing so I am reminded of Winston Churchill's famous declaration after Britain's long-awaited triumph at the 1942 Battle of El Alamein. It was the Allies' very first victory in World War II after an extended series of demoralizing defeats. Seizing the moment, Churchill announced to the world, "This is not the end. It is not even the beginning of the end. But it is, perhaps, the end of the beginning."

Acknowledgments

I am fortunate to have received much guidance and support in the course of my life and career. Writing this book was no exception. My greatest debt is to my parents, Howard and Ruth, whose love and influence formed my values, moral posture, and view of the world, and to my wife, Rosemarie, and sons, Jonathan and Jeremy, who have enriched my life immeasurably, supported my efforts, and graciously tolerated my many absences from them and family life as a result of my chronic overinvolvement with my professional activities (otherwise known as "workaholism").

When I first thought seriously about writing this book, Jim Shinn, a dear friend and professor of political economy and international relations at Princeton, helped me to crystallize the nub of the story from an inchoate conglomeration of ideas. He also pointed me in the direction of oncologist and fellow Columbia faculty member Siddhartha Mukherjee, who was kind enough to spend an illuminating hour with me. I have looked to Sid's Pulitzer Prize–winning book, *The Emperor of All Maladies*, as a model and a source of inspiration.

With a plan in mind, I sought advice from friends who also happen to be brilliant writers. Kay Jamison, Oliver Sacks, and Andrew Solomon offered encouragement, guided my formative thinking about the content, and helped me to navigate the publishing landscape and process. Peter Kramer gave helpful advice as a psychiatrist writing for the general public.

I owe thanks to my friend and neighbor Jennifer Weis, an editor at St. Martin's Press, who introduced me to my agent, Gail Ross of the Ross-Yoon Agency. Gail took the idea I pitched to her, expertly fashioned it into something more accessible, and connected me to Ogi Ogas, a skilled writer and neuroscientist. Ogi and I bonded and became virtual Siamese twins for the next eighteen months while developing the story and creating the manuscript. His invaluable contributions and unwavering dedication to the project were apparent throughout, but never more dramatically than when he convinced his fiancée to postpone their honeymoon so that he could finish the book with me on time.

Numerous colleagues generously gave me their time and provided valuable information during the research process, including Nancy Andreasen, the eminent researcher and professor of psychiatry at the University of Iowa; Aaron Beck, inventor of cognitive-behavioral therapy (CBT) and emeritus professor of psychiatry at the University of Pennsylvania; Bob Spitzer, the chair of *DSM-III* and emeritus professor of psychiatry at Columbia University, who, along with his wife and *DSM-III* Task Force member Janet Williams, recounted their experience with *DSM* and the evolution of psychiatry; Jean Endicott and Michael First, Columbia University faculty who worked with Spitzer and on various *DSM*s; Robert Innis, eminent scientist and chief of molecular imaging at the National Institute of Mental Health, who advised on the impact of imaging on psychiatry; Robert Lifton, psychiatrist-activist-author and Columbia University faculty member, who described his Vietnam-era experience and collaboration with Chaim Shatan; Bob Michels, the former dean of Cornell Medical College and eminent psychiatrist and psychoanalytic scholar, who, in erudite fashion, recounted the trajectory of psychoanalysis in American psychiatry; Roger Peele, the iconoclastic former chair of psychiatry at St. Elizabeths Hospital, in Washington, DC, and longstanding leader in the American Psychiatric Association, who shared his firsthand experience with the passage of *DSM-III*; Harold Pincus, former director of research of the APA and vice chair of *DSM-IV*, who provided an informative perspective on the APA and *DSM*; Myrna Weissman, the eminent psychiatric epidemiologist and professor of psychiatry at Columbia University, who described how she and her late husband, Gerry Klerman, developed Interpersonal Psychotherapy. Tim Walsh and Paul Appelbaum, eminent psychiatrists and Columbia professors, provided feedback on selected portions of the manuscript. Glenn Martin was the APA Assembly liaison to the *DSM-5* Task Force and helped me recall the chronology of events in the development process. Brigitt Rok, a friend and clinical psychologist, provided feedback on sections of the manuscript from the practitioner's perspective. My friend and colleague Wolfgang Fleischhacker, chair of biological psychiatry at the University of Innsbruck, enlightened me about historical developments in German and Austrian psychiatry, and translated key documents from German to English.

Hannah Decker's scholarly book *The Making of DSM-III: A Diagnostic Manual's Conquest of American Psychiatry* provided an invaluable source of information.

Four luminaries generously took the time to review large sections of the manuscript in various drafts and provide detailed comments. Andrew Solomon offered wise but bracing feedback in his review of an early version that got us started on the right track. Eric Kandel, the celebrated scientist, author, and Nobel laureate who is a university professor at Columbia, engaged in several discussions with me about psychiatry, past and present, and gave me relevant materials and valuable comments on sections of the manuscript. Both Fuller Torrey, the researcher, author, and public commentator and advocate for the mentally ill, and Ken Kendler, the renowned geneticist, scholar, and professor of psychiatry at Virginia Commonwealth University, spent lengthy periods reviewing near complete drafts of the manuscript and providing detailed feedback.

I also want to recognize Peter Zheutlin, a science writer who helped me on an earlier project that contributed to this book, and the journalist Stephen Fried, a member of the Columbia Journalism School faculty, who offered sage advice on effective writing for nonprofessional audiences.

Thanks to Michael Avedon, Annette Swanstrom, and Eve Vagg for taking and providing photos for the book. Yvonne Cole and Jordan DeVylder provided research assistance, and Yvonne and Monica Gallegos obtained permissions for photos and quotes used in the book. And, perhaps most important, Susan Palma and Monica Gallegos actively managed my schedule to block time for me to write the book.

When my agent and I first approached potential publishers, Tracy Behar, now my editor, responded with unabashed enthusiasm (along with the publisher Reagan Arthur) and preemptively engaged us with Little, Brown. Over the course of the book's development, Tracy, with the help of her associate Jean Garnett, guided us with skill and experience. Their timely and incisive comments and suggestions helped craft the book into its final form and length.

Finally, I want to acknowledge and express my gratitude to my teachers, mentors, psychiatric and scientific colleagues, and mental health care providers for what they have taught me, and the experiences I have enjoyed, and for their efforts to advance our knowledge of, and care for, people with mental illness. Like everything that we collectively do, this book is motivated by the desire to improve the lives of people with mental illness. I am grateful to my patients for the lessons that they have imparted to me, and the purpose that they have given to my life.

Sources and Additional Reading

Adler, A. *The Neurotic Constitution*. Translated by J. E. Lind and B. Glueck. New York: Moffat, Yard and Company, 1917.

Amen, D. G. *Change Your Brain, Change Your Life: The Breakthrough Program for Conquering Anxiety, Depression, Obsessiveness, Anger, and Impulsiveness*. New York: Three Rivers Press, 1998.

American Psychiatric Association. *Diagnostic and Statistical Manual of Mental Disorders: DSM-5*. 5th Edition. Washington, DC: American Psychiatric Publishing, 2013.

———. *The Statistical Manual for the Use of Institutions for the Insane, 1918*. New York: State Hospitals Press, 1942.

Beck, J. S., and A. T. Beck. *Cognitive Behavior Therapy, Second Edition: Basics and Beyond*. New York: The Guilford Press, 2011.

Boller, F., and G. D. Barba. "The Evolution of Psychiatry and Neurology: Two Disciplines Divided by a Common Goal?" In *Current Clinical Neurology: Psychiatry for Neurologists*, edited by D. V. Jeste and J. H. Friedman, 11–15. Totowa, NJ: Humana Press, 2006.

Brown, H. G. *Sex and the Single Girl: The Unmarried Woman's Guide to Men, 1962*. New York: Open Road Media, 2012.

Campbell, J. *The Hero with a Thousand Faces*. 3rd edition. Novato, CA: New World Library, 2008.

Castaneda, C. *The Teachings of Don Juan: A Yaqui Way of Knowledge*. Berkeley, CA: University of California Press, 1998.

Centonze, D., A. Siracusano, P. Calabresi, and G. Bernardi. "The 'Project for a Scientific Psychology' (1895): A Freudian Anticipation of LTP-Memory Connection Theory." *Brain Research Reviews* 46 (2004): 310–14.

Clarke, C. A., and P. M. Sheppard. "Lessons of the 'Pink Spots.'" *British Medical Journal* 1 (1967): 382–83.

Darwin, C. *On the Origin of Species by Means of Natural Selection*. London: John Murray Albemarle Street Publishers, 1859.

Decker, H. S. *The Making of DSM-III: A Diagnostic Manual's Conquest of American Psychiatry*. New York: Oxford University Press, 2013.

Diagnostic and Statistical Manual of Mental Illness. American Psychiatric Association Task Force on Nomenclature and Statistics. Washington, DC: American Psychiatric Publishing, 1952.

Dickstein, L. J., M. B. Riba, and J. M. Oldham, eds. *American Psychiatric Press Review of Psychiatry*. Washington, DC: American Psychiatric Press, 1997.

Dukakis, K. D. *Shock: The Healing Power of Electroconvulsive Therapy*. New York: Avery Publishing Group, 2006.

Ellenberger, H. *The Discovery of the Unconscious: The History and Evolution of Dynamic Psychiatry*. New York: Basic Books, Perseus Books Group, 1970.

Ellman, G. L., R. T. Jones, and R. C. Rychert. "Mauve Spot and Schizophrenia." *American Journal of Psychiatry* 125 (1968): 849–51.

Endler, J. A. "Gene Flow and Population Differentiation." *Science* 179 (1973): 243–50.

Feighner, J. P., E. Robins, S. B. Guze, A. Woodruff Jr., G. Winokur, and R. Munoz. "Diagnostic Criteria from the Saint Louis School (Missouri-USA)." *Archives of General Psychiatry* 26, no. 1 (1972): 57–63.

Feuchtersleben, E. von. *Principles of Medical Psychology*. London: Sydenham Society, 1847.

Frances, A. *Saving Normal: An Insider's Revolt Against Out-of-Control Psychiatric Diagnosis, DSM-5, Big Pharma and the Medicalization of Ordinary Life*. New York: HarperCollins, 2013.

Freedman, A. M., and H. I. Kaplan. *The Comprehensive Textbook of Psychiatry*. Baltimore, MD: Williams and Wilkins, 1967.

Freud, S. *Introductory Lectures on Psychoanalysis*. New York: Edward L. Bernays, Inc., 1920.

———. *Project for a Scientific Psychology*. In *The Complete Letters of Sigmund Freud to Wilhelm Fliess, 1887–1904*. Edited and translated by J. M. Masson. Cambridge, MA: Belknap Press of Harvard University Press, 1985.

———. *The Future of an Illusion*. Translated by G. C. Richter. Peterborough, Ontario, Canada: Broadview Press, 2012.

———. *The Interpretation of Dreams*. New York: The Macmillan Company, 1913.

———. *Totem and Taboo*. Translated by A. A. Brill. New York: Moffat, Yard and Company, 1918.

Gay, Peter. *Freud: A Life for Our Time*. New York: W. W. Norton and Company, 1988.

Goffman E. *Asylums*. New York: Doubleday and Company, 1961.

Gorwitz, K. "Census Enumeration of the Mentally Ill and the Mentally Retarded in the Nineteenth Century." *Health Service Report* 89, no. 2 (1974): 180–87.

Houts, A. C. "Fifty Years of Psychiatric Nomenclature: Reflections on the 1943 War Department Technical Bulletin, *Medical 203*." *Journal of Clinical Psychology* 56, no. 7 (2000): 953–67.

Hurn, J. D. "The History of General Paralysis of the Insane in Britain, 1830 to 1950." PhD diss., University of London, 1998.

Huxley, A. *The Doors of Perception: And Heaven and Hell.* New York: Vintage Classic, 2004.

Hyman, S. E., and E. J. Nestler. *The Molecular Foundations of Psychiatry.* Washington DC: American Psychiatric Press, 1993.

James, W. *The Varieties of Religious Experience.* Rockville, MD: Manor, 2008.

Jamison, K. R. *An Unquiet Mind: A Memoir of Moods and Madness.* New York: Vintage Books, 1996.

Jones, E., and S. Wessely. *Shell Shock to PTSD: Military Psychiatry from 1900 to the Gulf War,* Maudsley Monographs #47. Hove, UK, and New York: Psychology Press, 2005.

Jung, C. G. *Studies in Word-Association.* Translated by M. D. Eder. New York: Moffat, Yard and Company, 1919.

Kandel, E. R. "Psychotherapy and the Single Synapse: The Impact of Psychiatric Thought on Neurobiological Research." *New England Journal of Medicine* 301, no. 19 (1979):1028–37.

———. *The Molecular Biology of Memory Storage: A Dialogue Between Genes and Synapses.* Monograph Reprint. *Les Prix Nobel 2000.* Stockholm, Sweden: Norstedts Tryckeri, 2001.

———. *Psychiatry, Psychoanalysis, and the New Biology of Mind.* Washington, DC: American Psychiatric Publishing, 2005.

———. *In Search of Memory: The Emergence of a New Science Mind.* New York: W. W. Norton & Company, 2006.

Kendler, K. S. "The Structure of Psychiatric Science." *American Journal of Psychiatry* 171, no. 9 (September 2014): 931–38.

Kraepelin, E. *Compendium der Psychiatrie.* Leipzig, Germany: Verlag von Ambr. Abel, 1983.

Kramer, P. D. *Listening to Prozac: A Psychiatrist Explores Antidepressant Drugs and the Remaking of the Self.* New York: Viking Penguin, 1993.

Lidz, T. *The Origin and Treatment of Schizophrenic Disorders.* New York: Basic Books, 1973.

Lifton, R. J. *Death in Life: Survivors of Hiroshima.* New York: Random House, 1968.

Linehan, M. M. *Skills Training Manual for Treating Borderline Personality Disorder.* New York: The Guilford Press, 1993.

Makari, G. *Revolution in Mind: The Creation of Psychoanalysis.* New York: HarperCollins, 2008.

Menninger, K. A. *The Vital Balance: The Life Process in Mental Health and Illness, 1963.* New York: Penguin Books, 1977.

———. "War Department Bulletin, *Medical 203*—Office of the Surgeon General, Army Service Forces: Nomenclature of Psychiatric Disorders and Reactions, 1943." *Journal of Clinical Psychology* 56, no. 7 (2000): 925–34.

Mesmer, F. A. *Dissertation on the Discovery of Animal Magnetism, 1779. Mesmerism: Being the Discovery of Animal Magnetism.* Translated by J. Bouleur. Lynnwood, WA: Holmes Publishing Group, 2005 (rev. ed.).

Michels, R. "Giants of Psychiatry." *American Board of Psychiatry and Neurology 75th Anniversary Celebration.* Lecture presented to the American Board of Psychiatry and Neurology (ABPN), September 26, 2009.

———. "Psychiatry and Psychoanalysis in the United States." *Philosophical Issues in Psychiatry III: The Nature and Sources of Historical Change.* Lecture conducted from University of Copenhagen, Denmark, May 10, 2013.

Nabokov, V. *Strong Opinions,* 1st Vintage International Edition. New York: Random House, 1990.

Noguchi, H., and J. W. Moore. "A Demonstration of Treponema Pallidum in the Brain in Cases of General Paralysis." *Journal of General Physiology* 17, no. 2 (1913): 232–38.

Oldham, J. M., and M. B. Riba, eds. *American Psychiatric Press Review of Psychiatry.* Vol. 13. Washington, DC: American Psychiatric Publishing, 1994.

Pauley, J. *Skywriting: A Life Out of the Blue.* New York: Ballantine Books, 2005.

Platt, M. *Storming the Gates of Bedlam: How Dr. Nathan Kline Transformed the Treatment of Mental Illness.* Dumont, NJ: DePew Publishing, 2012.

Porter, R. *The Greatest Benefit to Mankind: A Medical History of Humanity.* New York: W. W. Norton & Company, 1999.

———. *Madness: A Brief History.* New York: Oxford University Press, 2002.

Protsch, R., and R. Berger. "Earliest Radiocarbon Dates for Domesticated Animals." *Science* 179 (1973): 235–39.

Rank, O. *The Trauma of Birth.* New York: Courier Dover Publications, 1929.

Reich, W. *The Function of the Orgasm: The Discovery of the Orgone.* V1. Rangeley, ME: The Orgone Institute Press, 1942.

Rollnick, S., W. R. Miller, and C. C. Butler. *Motivational Interviewing in Health Care: Helping Patients Change Behavior.* New York: The Guilford Press, 2008.

Rosenhan, D. L. "On Being Sane in Insane Places." *Science* 179 (January 1973): 250–58.

Rossner, J. *Looking for Mr. Goodbar.* New York: Washington Square Press, 1975.

Rush, B. *Medical Inquiries and Observations Upon the Diseases of the Mind.* Vols. 1–4. 2nd ed. Philadelphia: J. Conrad and Company, 1805.

Sacks, O. *Musicophilia: Tales of Music and the Brain.* New York: Alfred A. Knopf, 2007.

Saks, E. R. *The Center Cannot Hold: My Journey Through Madness.* New York: Hyperion Press, Hachette Publishing Group, 2007.

Scott, W. "PTSD in *DSM-III*: A Case in the Politics of Diagnosis and Disease." *Social Problems* 37, no. 3 (1990): 294–310.

Shephard, B. *A War of Nerves: Soldiers and Psychiatrists in the Twentieth Century.* Cambridge, MA: Harvard University Press, 2001.

Shorter, E. *A History of Psychiatry: From the Era of the Asylum to the Age of Prozac.* New York: John Wiley & Sons, 1997.

———. *A Historical Dictionary of Psychiatry.* New York: Oxford University Press, 2005.

Skinner, B. F. *Walden 2.* Indianapolis: Hackett Publishing Company, Inc., 1948.

Solomon, A. *Far from the Tree: Parents, Children and the Search for Identity.* New York: Simon & Schuster, 2012.

———. *The Noonday Demon: An Atlas of Depression.* New York: Scribner, 2003.

Spiegel, A. "The Dictionary of Disorder: How One Man Revolutionized Psychiatry." *The New Yorker,* January 3, 2005.

Steiner, M. A. "PET—the History behind the Technology." Master's thesis, University of Tennessee, Knoxville, TN, 2002.

Szasz, T. S. *The Myth of Mental Illness: Foundations of a Theory of Personal Conduct.* New York: HarperCollins 50th Anniversary Edition, 2011.

Torrey, F. E. *American Psychosis: How the Federal Government Destroyed the Mental Illness Treatment System.* New York: Oxford University Press, 2014.

———. *Freudian Fraud: The Malignant Effect of Freud's Theory on American Thought and Culture.* New York: Harper Collins, 1992.

———. *The Invisible Plague: The Rise of Mental Illness from 1750 to the Present,* with Judy Miller. Brunswick, NJ: Rutgers University Press, 2002.

———. *Nowhere to Go: The Tragic Odyssey of the Homeless Mentally Ill.* New York: Harper Collins, 1988.

———. *Out of the Shadows: Confronting America's Mental Illness Crisis.* New York: John Wiley & Sons, 1996.

War Department Bulletin, *Medical 203*—Office of the Surgeon General, Army Service Forces. "Nomenclature of Psychiatric Disorders and Reactions." *Journal of Clinical Psychology* 56, no. 7 (2000): 925–34.

Ward, M. J. *The Snake Pit.* New York: Random House, 1946.

Weissman M. M., J. C. Markowitz, and J. C. Klerman. *Comprehensive Guide to Interpersonal Psychotherapy.* New York: Basic Books, Perseus Books Group, 2000.

Wikipedia https://en.wikipedia.org/wiki/Main_Page.

Zubin, J. "Cross-National Study of Diagnosis of the Mental Disorders: Methodology and Planning." *American Journal of Psychiatry* 125 (1969): 12–20.

Copyright Acknowledgments

Index

About the Author

Jeffrey A. Lieberman, MD, has spent his career of over thirty years caring for patients and studying the nature and treatment of mental illness. Dr. Lieberman is the Lawrence C. Kolb Professor and Chairman of Psychiatry at the Columbia University College of Physicians and Surgeons and Director of the New York State Psychiatric Institute. He also holds the Lieber Chair for Schizophrenia Research in the Department of Psychiatry at Columbia and serves as Psychiatrist in Chief at New York Presbyterian Hospital–Columbia University Medical Center. His work has advanced our knowledge of the history and treatment of psychotic disorders and has fundamentally contributed to the current standards of care as well as the development of novel therapeutic medications and transformative strategies for the early detection and prevention of schizophrenia.

Dr. Lieberman has authored more than five hundred articles published in the scientific literature and has edited or coedited twelve books on mental illness and psychiatry. He is the recipient of many honors and awards, including the Lieber Prize for Schizophrenia Research from the Brain and Behavior Research Association, the Adolph Meyer Award from the American Psychiatric Association, the Stanley R. Dean Award for Schizophrenia Research from the American College of Psychiatry, the Research Award from the National Alliance on

Mental Illness, and the Neuroscience Award from the International College of Neuropsychopharmacology. Formerly the president of the American Psychiatric Association, he is a member of numerous scientific organizations and in 2000 was elected to the National Academy of Sciences Institute of Medicine.

He lives with his wife in New York City.